The Encyclopaedia of Celtic Reiki Essences

By
Martyn Pentecost

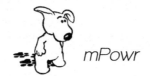

mPowr

First Published in Great Britain 2010 by mPowr (Publishing) Limited
www.mpowrpublishing.com
www.celtic-reiki.com

A catalogue record for this book is available from the British Library
ISBN – 978-1-907282-39-3

Cover Design by Martyn Pentecost
mPowr Publishing 'Clumpy™' Logo by e-nimation.com
Clumpy™ and the Clumpy™ Logo are trademarks of mPowr Limited

MADE BY BOOK BROWNIES!

Books published by mPowr Publishing are made by Book Brownies. A Book Brownie is about so high, with little green boots, a potato-like face and big brown eyes. These helpful little creatures tenderly create every book with kindness, care and a little bit of magic! Before shipping, a Book Brownie will jump into the pages—usually at the most gripping chapter or a part that pays particular attention to food—and stay with that book, always. This means that every mPowr Publishing book comes with added enchantment (and occasional chocolate smudges!) so that you get a warm, fuzzy feeling of love with the turn of every page!

Join us on the
Celtic Reiki Mastery Adventure...

Free Mastery Training
with this book.*

www.celtic-reiki.com

The only division we have is perspective…

CONTENTS

An Introduction to Essences

Energy is rather like the potential of a blank page; many would view the page simply as nothingness, whereas others would see amazing possibilities. On this simple canvas, we can write, sketch, paint, fold; we have the ability to create whatever we can imagine. Through the expressions that are placed on the page, we can share everything, through words, images, shapes and colours – a page will even soak up perfumes and flavours so that we have the opportunity to convey smell and taste sensations.

The essential aspect of this page is that to actually create some action (or reaction) it requires definition. A single line or fold gives definition; a word or even a smudge provides us with something that wasn't there before: identity.

Many people create identity of the page through cutting it up into smaller and smaller pieces, feeling this is the way to define something from nothing. I personally prefer to keep the page intact, but to create layering. By doing so, we have a page that can convey anything we want it to; all we need do is look at it from different angles or perspectives to make a change in what we sense.

This is the foundation of the essence—a definition of energy that is based on perspective, as opposed to separation. The value of this simple change of terminology and viewpoint is utterly breathtaking, because by changing our way of perceiving energy from the 'energies' of different 'flavour' or type, to the concept of energy as an all-encompassing force or potential, we embrace one vital aspect to the philosophy – the self. If you see energy as divided, or through the dynamic of separation, you become that dynamic and separate yourself from the oneness.

Imagine for a moment, somebody who is experiencing hatred for another. As they experience that emotion, they are physically, chemically and mentally 'in' that emotional state. The physiological actions of hatred are actively wrecking that person's health and well-being, clouding their thoughts and shifting their focus to the place where they take action, based on hatred. This not only gives them the results of those actions to deal with (results that can last a lifetime in some cases), but it also forms habitual responses and presents the person with 'evidence' that supports their perspective of the world. Our outlook has to be true in the world—if anything goes against what we believe, we distort or delete it to ensure we maintain our own 'truth'. Our example of a person hating, shows us that will often ignore instances where hate is inappropriate, in favour of more reasons to hate. Very often, the only thing that will release that person from hatred is time – as time passes, emotions fade and a person's 'filters' can change.

This is exactly the same process for separation; a person who uses the filters of division through separation (cutting the paper up) is in that dynamic. The 'shape' of separation fills their life and affects their actions, clouds thoughts, and offers more examples of a world divorced and separate from them.

Therefore, when you approach this new perspective (of unity and fluidity), your existing filters may kick-in and attempt to resist this new way of thinking. The challenge would be that society is expanding outwards from isolation to integration, from separation to unity. This expansion is powered by the strength of momentum (an incomprehensible, unstoppable force when applied to the progression of humankind).

The old resistances of the 'separation mentality' could shift you out of flow and cause contraction—you are oneness, expanding towards self-realisation; thus the creation of barriers and boundaries creates internal pain, rather than the joy of flow.

The greatest challenge of Mastery is the letting-go of old habits, redefinition of oneself, and the ability to step into a new way of perceiving the Universe. Celtic Reiki, as an adaptive system of personal development, invites us to expand beyond separation and isolation to view our practice as a method for creating unity and oneness. We are always striving to integrate through the definition of context and perspective, so that every individual remains a part of the whole; the complex dance of life and conscious experience.

Essences provide us with a way of understanding the entire Universe—everything that ever was, is, or will be – defined from a single perspective: that of a tree, species of tree, rock, or concept. Thus essences open up a whole new way of viewing the way we comprehend Celtic Reiki, because with the philosophy of essences, we:

- Shift our own perspective, as opposed to 'changing energy'
- Maintain connection/oneness between the definitions of Master, client, and energy
- Can work with people from all layers of social dynamics, and actually expand our own social dynamics in the process (see The Adventurer's Guide for further information)
- Attain fluidity of treatment and practice, personal development and global change
- Present a smoother transition for clients and ourselves, between perspectives (the perspective of dis-ease to the perspective of health, for example – it is easier to 'change one's mind' than to 'recover from illness')
- Instil a greater confidence in students, as the system becomes rooted in 'personal perspective', rather than the right/wrong way of doing things
- Achieve a greater ease of learning, because Orientation and Calibration suggests a simple change of viewpoint, as distinct from having to do some impossible, mystical task (some people like the challenge of the mystical task and if you are one of these people, I recommend you think about the spiritual beauty and conundrum of a single thought, versus a complex ritual)

These are but a few of the benefits an 'essence philosophy' offers us in practice and Mastery, and in many ways, I understand the change of ethos to be more about what I have yet to learn, as opposed to my current knowledge. If I have grasped one thing along the way, it would be to make room for what I don't yet know; for when I trust the shaping abilities of the intelligences I work with, there is always a perfect fit just a little way into the future!

What follows is a framework; a vast range of perspectives that can be shifted and shaped to your own view and practice. And herein lies the real power of the essence, because if I were to present you with a selection of different 'types' or 'flavours' of energy, these would come with predefined principles, 'rules' and specific areas of use. The perspective, however, naturally differs from person to person; so what I offer you, in fact, is a foundation that is flexible enough to be adapted.

Through the testing process, I have collated the common themes of my own clients' feedback and my experiences of harvesting and teaching these essences. It is a gift that I offer, for you to take and make your own— to shape and mould, to adapt and alter, or even to change completely if your own experiences in practice presents you with different feedback.

Our own common sense tells us that it is possible to see a tree, brightly lit by sunshine, whilst another sees the same tree at the same time, in silhouette; it all depends on definition, position, and perception. The same is true of all essences and definitions of energy that do not involve the 'cutting of the page', as this is the process of making energy 'permanent' and is akin to filming a tree bathed in sunlight and then using that as a Universal truth that the tree cannot be in shadow!

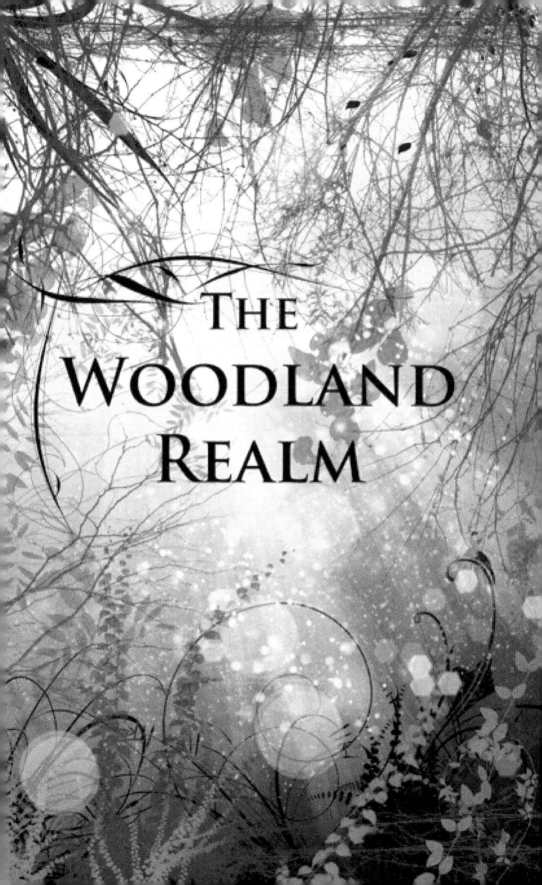

The
Woodland
Realm

THE
CELTIC TREE
ESSENCES

Ailim

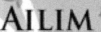

Pine, Fir, Spruce and Conifer
A - [ARLM]

Once Upon a Time...

...THERE WAS A TREE WHO WAS GIVEN THE TASK OF GUARDIANSHIP. HIS POSITION WAS TO KEEP THE OTHER TREES OF THE FOREST OUT OF THE GRASP OF THE BURNING WIND. HE KNEW THAT TO COMPLETE HIS TASK, HE WOULD NEED TO GROW TALLER THAN EVERY OTHER TREE IN THE FOREST, SO EACH AND EVERY DAY HE STRIVED MORE THAN ANY OTHER TREE TO BE THE TALLEST. AND BEFORE HE KNEW IT, HE COULD SEE RIGHT ACROSS THE FOREST, PAST ALL THE OTHER TREES, TO THE HORIZON IN EVERY DIRECTION.

IT WASN'T LONG BEFORE THE OTHER TREES AND THE DWELLERS OF THE WOODLAND REALM ASKED EACH DAY, WHAT HE COULD SEE. HE WOULD TELL THEM STORIES OF FARAWAY PLACES, BEYOND THE BOUNDARIES OF THE FOREST. GRADUALLY, PASSING TRAVELLERS AND THOSE WITH NO PLACE TO GO GATHERED TO LISTEN TO HIS TALES AND SOON, CLIMBED INTO HIS BRANCHES TO SHELTER FROM THE ELEMENTS AS THEY REVELLED IN THE FANTASTIC SIGHTS THAT THE TREE SPOKE ABOUT.

IT CAME TO PASS THAT THIS TREE AND HIS KIND WERE NAMED 'AILIM', THE GIVER OF SIGHT, THE GUARDIAN, THE HOME TO THOSE THAT HAVE NO HOME...

Ailim is of the Silver Fir, the Pine, the Spruce and the Conifer – he helps to clarify vision and to see the way forward (the horizon). Ailim breaks down barriers to the lessons learnt over our life-time; increasing wisdom from the past, increasing the connection to Celtic Wisdom and binding this to our consciousness, thus solving current issues in a person's life.

The essence is particularly useful in looking to the very distant future, in areas such as life goals or life's work and helps integrate a person with their purpose. It can also connect the user to their Celtic ancestry if relevant.

Physical: Of particular use on the mucus membrane and for clearing the nasal and respiratory tracts. Also has been seen to be very effective on any condition of the bladder and urinary tract.

Emotional/Mental: Lack of vision – cannot see a worthwhile future. Ailim is excellent for those who are unaware of or deny their qualities and achievements. Guilt and self-reproach are other areas where Ailim can be of use. Fear and loss, especially loss of one's home (being uprooted or cut off from one's roots). For the explorer, the nomad and the migrant, Ailim gives comfort and creates a sense of home, wherever you are.

Spiritual: Spiritual Vision - a finding of a life path and awakening of psychic/intuitive abilities. For spiritual development and a widening of perspective on spiritual matters.

The Message of Ailim

I help those who are lost and cannot find their way in the darkness—I am sight, I am vision, I am home. For those who have been hurt in terrible, sometimes near fatal ways I can bring peace and understanding to what cannot be understood. For those who have lost their homes or who have been forced to leave their countries and homelands, I offer sanctuary and the ability to live in new places and circumstances.

I can be the comfort needed wherever there is death and destruction. In war, I offer peace, and in heartache I offer healing. For those who have striven for many years on paths that have led them to dead ends or perceived failure, I suggest new perspectives and alternative ways forward.

I offer healing to the sick in all physical disease, pain and loss—especially where something has been lost such as a limb or after major surgery to remove diseased aspects of the body. I have an affinity with children who are unwell and suffering in physical and emotional pain; including those who have been so ill in their short life that it will affect them into adulthood or may even take them prematurely. I soothe those who have lost one or more of their parents and those who have suffered great trauma as children. I heal the pain inflicted by humankind on its fellows and the abuse that is done by one individual to another—both male and female.

I support those who have been attacked or raped, whether they are male or female and regardless of the gender of the abuser. I create strength and complete reconciliation where there has been 'violation'.

I see all. I can guide you to a place where you are healed and completely loved. Even when you can see no path, no way forward, no hope, I am there standing above all others—so look to the horizon and see the tall, wise Spruce tree that stands proud and defiant against all pain and abuse: that is me. I am Ailim.

THE ORACLE OF AILIM

When the Ailim weaves his magic into a reading, you are asked to think back to the past or forward to the future and how these fragments of time play an important role in the present; as lessons you have learnt or experiences that are yet to come.

If you are in a situation where you cannot seem to break away from some past event or trauma; if your memories hold you back; if the experiences you have encountered to this point create a fear that seems to prevent you from being all you can be, the Ailim Essence is here to help. For the challenges that you have survived have made you strong. The actual circumstances are gone in the physical world and only their memory remains – thus the situation cannot actually hurt you anymore.

Ailim encourages you to learn from the hurts of the past so that you never have to experience these again. The strength you gained from traversing these painful experiences will act as a shepherd for the current situation and will guide you through the darkness—to a brighter and happier place. Ailim beckons you forward to the unknown, explaining that the past can be your prison or your liberation, depending on how you use it. The Ailim essence also represents intuition and the ability to see beyond your senses – to experience the future with the ability to nurture or change what you're currently manifesting in your life.

Ailim can signify a journey or travel to another place, especially that to faraway places in a migratory sense of emigration to another country or long term moving to home that is different from where you are currently based. This journey may be of the physical world, and yet, could also denote an emotional, cerebral or spiritual journey to another state of consciousness or perspective of life.

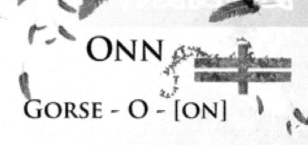

ONN

GORSE - O - [ON]

THERE ONCE WAS A LITTLE BIRD

THAT WAS CHASED ACROSS THE REALMS BY A GROUP OF MAGPIES, WHO TEASED AND TORMENTED HER UNTIL SHE HAD NO STRENGTH LEFT WITH WHICH TO GO ON. SO SHE FELL TO EARTH, WHERE A HANDSOME, YOUNG TREE CAUGHT HER IN HIS BRANCHES.

"WHAT IS WRONG?" HE ASKED THE BIRD, WHO IN RETURN, TOLD THE TREE OF HER PLIGHT. "I WILL PROTECT YOU FROM THE MAGPIES!" HE PROMISED, AS HE WRAPPED HER UP IN HIS LEAVES, TO SLEEP, TO DREAM.

FOR MANY YEARS THE TREE KEPT THE LITTLE BIRD SAFE, HOWEVER, THE MAGPIES WERE CUNNING AND SOON DISCOVERED CLEVER WAYS OF DECEIVING THE TREE. SO HE DECIDED TO GET CREATIVE IN HIS APPROACH. FIRST OF ALL HE GREW BEAUTIFUL, YELLOW FLOWERS THAT SCENTED THE AIR WITH COCONUT BUTTER. THE BEES FOLLOWED THE SWEET AROMA TO HIS FLOWERS WHERE THEY DRANK SWEET NECTAR AND STUNG THE MAGPIES IF THEY GOT TOO CLOSE.

WHEN THE WINTER CAME, HOWEVER THE BEES WENT TO SLEEP AND THE FLOWERS FADED AWAY, SO THE TREE GREW LONG, SHARP THORNS TO WARD AWAY THE MAGPIES, WHO COULD NOT PENETRATE THE WILD AND PAINFUL GROWTH OF THE TREE, TO GET TO THE LITTLE BIRD, SAFE AND WARM INSIDE. THIS TREE BECAME KNOWN TO THOSE IN THE WOODLAND REALM AS ONN; CREATIVE THINKER AND DEFENDER OF THE WEAK...

The Gorse creates a gathering of inner strength to help those who feel weak or unable to cope, filling them with renewed vigour; tapping into their own source of power and joy so that it empowers them in the future.

Gorse is a remarkable creature, for he possesses such fearsome and numerous thorns and yet is capable of such beauty. Onn seems to mirror so many people in our world, for his need to assert himself has created the thorns that drive many away, yet he proclaims his need for love with the beautiful flowers that shine like gold on a summer's day, filling the air with sweet scent.

He says, "Come gaze upon my beauty, breathe in my heavenly scent, and touch me softly, but do not get too close as I will hurt you!"

In actual fact, the Gorse is not nearly as formidable as he may appear upon first inspection, for although he does have a barrage of thorns; he is a very gentle tree. I have reached out to touch Gorse plants during howling gales and they seem to stop their thrashing at the place where you touch them, almost as if they hold strong against the wind, so as not to cause you harm.

Gorse offers protection to much of the local wildlife, providing shelter in places that are often inhospitable or prone to extreme weather. The beautiful yellow flowers offer abundant nectar to the insects, carpeting hills, valleys and moors with such vibrant beauty as to take one's breath away.

Onn works with the building of inner strength helping those who feel weak or unable to cope with renewed vigour; tapping them into their own source of strength and joy so that it lasts and empowers them in the future.

The Celts are believed to have viewed the Onn Essence as being a very innovative essence, used to stimulate the creative juices, nurture new ways of thinking, develop artistic ability and otherwise push the personal evolutionary process forward.

The beautiful outlook of Onn sparkles with colour and light, awakening the senses and giving a heightened perception of the world, enabling us to experience our lives through many different sensory experiences, in addition to the five senses that are usually used.

Onn provides colour to those who only see in black and white, allowing them to experience the joy of coming from a monochrome world to one of brilliant Technicolor.

The essence of Onn is also wonderful at producing a balanced view of the black and the white for those who only want the colourful aspects of life. For instance, when dealing with people who sacrifice their spiritual journey or life path for the sake of hedonism, physical pleasure, materialism, addiction, etc. Onn reminds us that the black and the white are there to protect us from our human nature and ourselves.

Physical: Help for those facing physical death. Works well in alleviating the symptoms of depression and side-effects of hormone imbalances.

Emotional/Mental: Helps people to come to terms with the emotional effects of terminal illness and a facing up to death of the physical. Brings out the creative spirit and helps artists/ performers connect to their own spark of inspiration. Onn assists with the gathering of inner strength to help those who feel weak or unable to cope. By providing us with renewed vigour, the Gorse taps us into our own source of strength and joy.

Spiritual: Restores faith for those who feel lost or have suffered some terrible trauma. Restores belief in the benevolence of source, life, and humankind.

THE ORACLE OF ONN

The Essence of Onn invites you to bring more passion into your life—from saturating everything you do with passion, to focussing more of your time on activities that you are passionate about.

There is a particular emphasis on creativity when this essence connects to your reading, so if you love being artistic, creating beauty, singing, dancing, playing or writing music, poetry, writing, or any other creative venture, Onn encourages you to give yourself time to explore these things with a full-on commitment.

Onn also denotes a lack of vibrancy in life—stagnation and of stuck in a rut. If you feel stuck in any aspect of your life, be it relationships, work, or some other part of your daily living, Onn is here to offer energy and potency to get you moving once again. This lack of vigour can also relate to a physical issue, involving a lack of energy, lethargy, tiredness and so on.

Maybe it is time to nurture yourself and set some boundaries that encompass your needs. Are you being walked over or taken advantage of?

Well, Onn is here to surround you with its defensive thorns and ward off any overbearing influence, aggression, or domineering force that you encounter, so that you can simply relax and recharge the soft, heady scent of coconut butter flowers and bright, yellow vibrancy—until you feel refreshed and ready to take on the world, once more!

If you are currently wondering about love, either a lack of love, a lack-lustre love, or the fading of love—Onn is a very positive sign of new love, rekindled love and a deepening of existing loving relationships.

The is a strength and depth to the emotion of Onn that will immerse you in the romance and passion of a loving relationship like never before, so be prepared for something or someone wonderful, just waiting to enter your life when you are ready to invite them in!

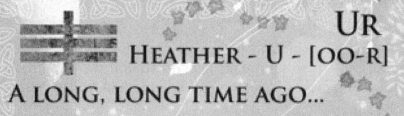

UR
HEATHER - U - [OO-R]

A LONG, LONG TIME AGO...

...WHEN THE TREES WHERE YOUNG AND NOT AS WISE AS THEY ARE NOW, THEY GORGED THEMSELVES ON THE TREASURES OF THE EARTH. EACH DAY THEY WOULD DRINK AND EAT AND SUCK THE VERY GROUND DRY OF WATER AND NUTRIENTS. THEY LAUGHED AND CARED FOR NOTHING BUT THEMSELVES. THEY GREW BIGGER AND FATTER, CLIMBING HIGH INTO THE SKY AND BECOMING COMPLETELY ADDICTED TO THEIR LAVISH WAYS.

THERE WAS, HOWEVER, ONE SMALL GROUP OF TREES THAT DID NOT TAKE MORE THAN THEY NEEDED. THESE TREES STAYED VERY SMALL AND DID NOT GET MUCH LIGHT ON THE FOREST FLOOR. YET, THEY SUNG AND THANKED THE EARTH EACH DAY; IN THEIR CONTENTMENT, THEY GREW LITTLE PINK AND WHITE FLOWERS AND WHEN THE OTHER TREES LAUGHED, THEY JUST SMILED SWEETLY AND WENT ABOUT THEIR BUSINESS.

SOON, THE EARTH GREW SO DRY THAT THE GROUND COULD NOT SUPPORT THESE MASSIVE, GREEDY TREES AND ONE BY ONE, THEY BEGAN TO DIE. WITHIN A FEW YEARS, MUCH OF THE ANCIENT FOREST WAS GONE AND ONLY SCRUBLAND OR MOOR WAS LEFT. NONETHELESS, THE LITTLE PINK AND WHITE TREES REMAINED, FOR THEY HAD POSSESSED THE WISDOM AND FORESIGHT TO ONLY TAKE WHAT THEY NEEDED AND NEVER TO BECOME DEPENDENT ON EXCESS. THE REMAINING TREES PUT THE SUCCESS OF THESE SMALL TREES DOWN TO LUCK AND THEREFORE, THEY CAME TO BE KNOWN AS UR; THOSE OF GOOD-FORTUNE AND WISDOM.

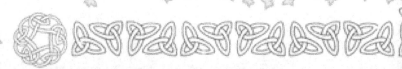

The Heather has been revered for centuries, particular the 'lucky' white heather that is so popular that it is now starting to disappear from the wild due to collection from those who wish to make use of its auspicious essence.

A greater understanding of the energetic nature of plants and trees offers us the wisdom that you do not need to uproot or harvest the physical being in order to work with the viewpoint it possesses.

The 'luck' essence of Ur assists us in the manifestation of our heaven on earth, as we strive towards a better life for all living things. Whether you believe in the random nature of luck as a concept or see luck as being an expression of being in 'flow', Ur will help you to realise your goals and bring the opportunities and necessary situations towards you.

By connecting us to the Earth and the natural world, Ur enables us to see our goal from a higher perspective. The essence also helps us to seek out the Deva and other forms of woodland entity who can guide us on the right way forward. This strengthening of connections to our unseen realms enables us to work with nature in an intuitive way, rather than analysing what we need to do. Thus we dissolve the barriers that we encounter and start to work with essences in a more integral way.

Excellent in manifestation and healing alike, Ur helps us to perceive the world in a very different way, whether it be helping us to attract prosperity, diluting our limiting beliefs towards money, discovering inner peace, calming the world around us, healing the diseased or healing the diseases within us.

The Ur essence was given to us by many different heather colonies that range in location across the British Isles, from Scotland, Wales, and various parts of England.

Physical: Diseases of the feet and ankles, especially fungal infections and issues with the soles of the feet, such as collapsed arches.

Emotional/Mental: Brings a sense of joy and prosperity into the heart and mind. Connects us to the true meaning of Wealth, not in a 'monetary' sense, but in the richness of life and happiness.

Spiritual: Tranquillity of the spirit and the sacred art of prophecy are both developed through use of Ur. Manifesting Heaven on Earth and connection to Deva of the woodland.

THE ORACLE OF UR

If you are interested in knowing more about the area of abundance in your current situation, then the essence of Ur is the one of the most joyous and positive layers of energy to pervade any reading.

Traditionally referred to as 'lucky' the heather has become synonymous with good fortune, prosperity and the upturn of any situation. This expansive and incredibly powerful essence displays the achievement of financial goals, the attainment of more money or greater income and proffers an overall sense of abundance in all things.

The revelations that Ur bring are numerous and plentiful, so treasure this vibrant essence and invite it into your perception, so that it may work its magic for you and those you love.

The connection to Ur in your reading today also favours games of chance such as the lottery and so on. Though remember that gambling in a monetary sense is not necessary when you have a truly abundant attitude, for when you ask from the perspective of wealth, the answer will find its way to you without the need to make bet or gamble.

The heather also signifies a general increase in fortunes and overall positivity in your life – prepare for a period of rapid growth and expansion as you become abundant in other area of your current situation—from happy occasions and good family relationships, to the daily joys of experience and sharing with others. As you enter this next phase of your life, you'll be amazed when you look around and see that you're surrounded by so much of what you desire that you'll be fit to burst with excitement!

If the Ur essence is appearing in the past – put your money to good use, spend wisely and invest. Show gratitude for what you have and have been given in the past and this will bring you more occasions for celebration in the future!

Eadha
Poplar and Aspen
E - [EE-YUR]

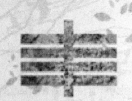

There once was a time...

...WHEN TREES FEARED DEATH AND DISEASE; THEY HAD YET TO LEARN OF THE CYCLES OF BIRTH AND REBIRTH, OF ONENESS AND UNITY THROUGH THE EARTH. IN THEIR FEAR, ISOLATION AND WORRY, TREES ADOPTED SOME RATHER UNUSUAL HABITS, FOR EXAMPLE: SOME WOULD ONLY GROW WHEN THOSE AROUND WERE TALLER, SO THAT THEY NEVER GOT MORE SUNLIGHT THAN THEIR NEIGHBOURS, OTHER TREES REFUSED TO GROW UNLESS EVERY SINGLE CONDITION WAS PERFECT, AND THERE WERE EVEN TREES THAT SIMPLY FOUND THEIR FEAR TOO MUCH TO COPE WITH SO THEY MANIFESTED THE VERY THING THAT SCARED THEM AND DIED.

THERE WERE A FEW TREES, HOWEVER, THAT LEARNT TO CONTROL THEIR FEAR, BUT PUTTING IT ON THE UNDERNEATH OF THEIR LEAVES. HENCE, TO LOOK AT THEM, YOU WOULD NEVER KNOW OF THEIR FEAR, BUT TURN OVER A LEAF AND YOU WOULD SEE PURE WHITE DUST – A SYMBOL OF THEIR FEAR BEING CONSTANTLY RELEASED. BY LETTING GO OF THEIR FEARS, THE EADHA LEARNED HOW TO LIVE WITH FEAR, WORRY AND ISOLATION IN A WAY THAT MEANT IT NEVER NEITHER HELD THEM BACK NOR STOPPED THEM FROM ENJOYING LIFE TO THE FULL.

Physical: Excellent for the nail, hair and scalp, as well as strengthening the teeth and cleansing the skin.

Emotional/Mental: Eadha helps to overcome fear: fear of the future, of responsibilities that may seem overwhelming; of the path we take and of the individual gifts we bring to the world. Eadha shields from the burden of the road ahead, helping us to work through and cope with the issues that may otherwise have pulled us down. This essence is excellent at helping when the pressures of life get too much and a person fears that they cannot cope with the world around them.

Spiritual: Eadha strengthens our spiritual resolve and gives us the ability to shout down the terrors we have with a whisper.

The Oracle of Eadha

In the essence of the popular, we uncover the darkness and the light—the inner world and the outer world. Yet these are not opposites—the darkness is not in polarity to the light; it is the lack of light! When you flick a light switch light appears, however, when you turn the light off, the darkness does not appear as the light does – the light disappears, revealing the darkness.

The essence of the Poplar is most powerful when in connected to the inner world of spiritual strength, emotional resolve, hidden potential, secret power, and undiscovered wisdom and the outer world of expansion into the new, spiritual tests, interpersonal experience and circumstances in the world around us. The appearance of this essence may signify some challenge to be overcome, or the inspiration to move forward.

It is at times of the greatest challenge when we discover our rare inner qualities and create opportunities to grow beyond our limitations—through adversity we learn to truly fly! Yet, this essence is not about adversity, it is about the transcendence of adversity.

If you have been experiencing pain, trauma, or dark times, you will soon find the answers you need to overcome these issues and step into better times, happier time, more vibrant and lighter times.

If you are currently in a stressful, busy and overwhelming situation, now is the time to step inside of oneself – you go inwards and spend time in the darkness—the serene, soft, all-compassing blackness of inner-peace and meditation.

There are answers within you—powerful portents of who you are and the person you can become if you are only willing to trust your inner strength.

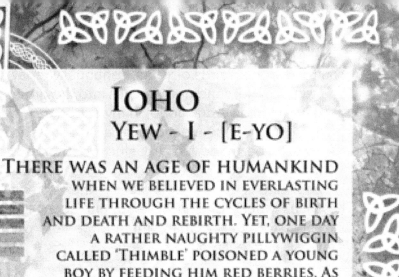

Ioho
Yew - I - [E-yo]

There was an age of humankind when we believed in everlasting life through the cycles of birth and death and rebirth. Yet, one day a rather naughty pillywiggin called 'Thimble' poisoned a young boy by feeding him red berries. As the boy lie dying, Thimble told him that this was a special poison that would send him to sleep forever. He would never be able to wake from his slumber and would never be reborn again.

This terrible deed of Thimble's was noticed by her twin brother, 'Fuddle' who was so upset by Thimble's actions that he called upon the Horned God, Cernunnos to come and help the lad. When the Lord of the Woodland came to see the boy, he was dismayed to see that to boy had slipped into his long sleep.

So, Cernunnos reached into the boy's tummy and touched the seeds of the red berries that began to grow inside of him. As the berries grew, the boy was transformed into a tree that would live for thousands of years. This tree was known as Ioho and he lived by constantly renewing himself, growing outwards and becoming hollow on the inside, so that the poison in his tummy could never harm him again. Consequently, Ioho and his offspring became associated with birth, death, and rebirth – reminding us that we live on through transformation and change.

The Yew Tree is the Celtic symbol of eternal life, as the Yew can live for thousands of years, continually renewing itself in an eternal cycle; sending branches into the ground that root, forming a hollow trunk. Ioho, in my experience, triggers one of the strongest connections of all the essences and was the first to be made into a Celtic Tree Remedy and Celtic Vibrational Remedy.

Ioho also helps increase the potency of other essences when used in a treatment and will cement the essences together to make them more fluid when acting in synthesis with each other.

Physical: Ioho can help in cases of poisoning and also helps with diseases of the very young or the very old. It has long been associated with death and therefore can help the physical passing of a person. Works well on the kidney and liver area.

Emotional/Mental: Ioho can help a person to "come back from the dead" on an emotional/mental level and so is good for issues such as nervous breakdowns, SDI, severe mental trauma.

Spiritual: The beginning and the end, the light and the dark. Ioho has the ability to resurrect spiritual faith that is lost and to bring what is hidden to the light. Used to treat eternal cycles that cannot be broken, or to create cycles that help a person to move forward – for example, those who cannot stick to any task, who are unable to motivate themselves or seem to be on an eternal path that gets them nowhere. Excellent for people who always make the same mistakes and never seem to learn or still create the same cycles even after learning the errors of their actions. Ioho helps increase the potency of other essences when used in a treatment and will also help cement the essences used in a forest to make them more fluid while acting in synthesis with each other.

THE ORACLE OF IOHO

The presence of Ioho may signify the next step in the cycle of birth—death—and rebirth. If you are planning a project or new phase in your life, the Yew denotes that a time of inception is rapidly approaching, when you will spread your wings and fly – your project or dreams will soon achieve enough momentum to become self-sufficient and take on a life of its own.

If you are currently running a project or have been striving for a long time with some element of your life, the Ioho essence is calling to you that it is time to let go and allow this particular chapter to reach its natural conclusion. The death cycle is often feared, however it is the ending of one thing that leads to the creation of another.

Is it time to reconsider your path, to make different choices, or to put old scores or issues to bed? Is it time to let go of the past and to move on? Is it time to say goodbye?

Don't worry, for immediately after death comes rebirth—the reinvention of the old into the new—the better—the superior! Like a phoenix from the ashes of what was, you will come anew and be more than you have ever been!

The Ioho essence also acts as a guardian or protector for those at peace. If you need time to yourself, to sit and ponder, to simply be, or to have the space to make important decisions, the Ioho essence will provide the necessary time and distance to shield you from the outside world and all your commitments, whilst you take the time you need.

A companion in times of need, the Yew tree whispers gently "I am here for you—do not be afraid, because I will guide and protect you!"

BEITH

BIRCH - B - [BEH]

THEY SAY, THERE WAS A TREE

WHO WOULD ONLY LIVE FOR EIGHTY YEARS, LOOKING BEAUTIFUL EACH AND EVERY DAY, BEFORE DISAPPEARING BACK INTO THE EARTH. IT WAS BECAUSE OF THIS NEWNESS THAT THEY CALLED HER BEITH; THE TREE OF BIRTH AND NEW BEGINNINGS. IN THE BEITH TONGUE THERE IS NO TIME FOR NEGATIVITY OR CONTRACTION INTO DESTRUCTIVE EMOTIONS – ONLY A MESSAGE OF HOPE AND FRESHNESS. FOR BEITH SEES THE WORLD ANEW IN EACH AND EVERY MOMENT, SHE KNOWS THAT ANYTHING IS POSSIBLE AND EVEN THE TOUGHEST CHALLENGE CAN BE MET AND OVERCOME IF YOU BELIEVE IT SO.

IN THE FIRST DAYS OF TREES, THERE WAS AN ANCESTOR OF BEITH, WHO ONLY SPOKE ILL AND NEVER SAW THE GOOD IN OTHERS. SHE WOULD SPEND EACH AND EVERY SUMMER FINDING FAULT AND BEING GENERALLY BAD TEMPERED. EVENTUALLY, NO SEED WOULD SPROUT NEAR HER AND NO BIRD WOULD SING, FOR FEAR OF BEING CHIDED OR CHASTISED BY THIS FEARSOME INDIVIDUAL.

THOUGH SOON, EIGHTY YEARS HAD BEEN AND GONE, AND THE OLD BEITH TREE REALISED HER TIME HAD COME. AS SHE STARTED TO CRUMPLE INTO THE GROUND, SHE WAS HEARD TO SAY ONE LAST THING... "IT'S ALL SO BEAUTIFUL AND I NEVER TOOK THE TIME TO NOTICE!"

HENCE, TO THIS DAY, ALL THE TREES THAT ARE BORN OF THE BEITH TONGUE WILL NEVER WASTE A MOMENT LOOKING FOR YUCK OR HORRIDNESS. THERE IS ONLY BEAUTY AND HOPE AND THE PROSPECT OF SOMETHING WONDERFUL TO COME...

Beith is of the Birch Tree and assists in the release of old ways, negative beliefs and reactions. She clears the past to make way for the present and the future, helps us to work through issues that are holding us back, cleansing and letting go.

She is also wonderful with helping to motivate at the start of a new venture. Often beginning something is the hardest thing to do - Beith will assist you in getting over any initial inertia in starting a new project.

Another side of Beith is that of forgiveness, helping us to forgive those who have hurt us in the past, she allows us to release any negative reactions we face.

The Birch is the initiator; the tree of new beginnings and fresh starts and is very relevant in our ever-changing and evolving world. I have worked with many birch trees over the years and have had the opportunity to meet many different individuals of other birch species, such as a magnificent 'paper birch' whose essence offers help and support to those who want to 'shed their old skin', or change in some integral way.

She also provides help for those with dry and flaky skin conditions such as psoriasis or eczema as well as helping ease the effects of flaky scalps and conditions of dryness/ dehydration.

The ability to help those who are starting anew after changing or are coming to terms with a fresh start after some major transition or loss has brought the Beith essence to a new level of effectiveness and created a greater integrity of the vibrations. This enables flexibility and rebirth as well as the processes of birth for the first time.

Physical: All skin conditions, muscular illness, or pain. It can be used as an appetite suppressant for those who wish to lose weight.

Emotional/Mental: Creates a feeling of newness and renewed optimism for the future. Clears the past to wipe the slate clean and offer fresh approaches to old problems. Motivator and energiser.

Spiritual: Renews spiritual growth and enables us to accept new concepts with ease.

THE ORACLE OF BEITH

The Birch is the tree of initiation and new beginnings, with the commencement of any new venture or project particularly well favoured. When Beith visits you in any reading the position of her arrival is of particular importance; for when she is in the past position, she is nudging you to proceed with projects that you have started, but not really developed as of yet.

In the present position, she murmurs that it is time to begin any new venture or adventure, as the energy if perfect at this time—go for it now! In the future position, Beith tells you to prepare for a new chapter in your life; being to gather resources, define and arrange your plans, because when the time comes to launch into this new phase, it will be all go—thus, the better prepared you can be, the easier it will be in the future.

Beith may bring news of the birth of a child, pregnancy and motherhood, along with a period of lifestyle change and moving on from pain and suffering. If you need to forgive somebody, or to forgive yourself for some past wrong, now is the time to do so, no matter how challenging it may seem.

The birch reminds us that holding on to anger and hate, keeps us immersed in those emotions, so for your own well-being, release the past and allow yourself the freedom of letting go.

Overcoming the inertia of a 'stuck', stalled, derailed project is also encompassed within this essence, as is initiation and the welcoming into a new group, family, relationship or circle of friends.

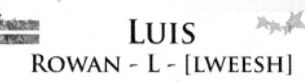

LUIS
ROWAN - L - [LWEESH]

A TREE ONCE STOOD

ATOP A LOFTY MOUNTAIN, WHERE
LIFE WAS COLD AND FULL OF FOREBODING. YET, NEVER A
DAY WENT BY THAT THE TREE DID NOT THANK THE
MOUNTAIN FOR HER HOSPITALITY, NOR WOULD HE EVER
TURN AWAY A LOST BIRD OR CREATURE FROM THE
SHELTER OF HIS BRANCHES. FOR THIS CHEERY CHAP
LOVED HIS TREACHEROUS, INHOSPITABLE HOME.

ONE COLD WINTER'S DAY THE GODDESS RHIANNON
WAS PASSING, WHEN SHE NOTICED THE LITTLE TREE
AND STOPPED TO ASK HIM WHY HE SEEMED DO HAPPY
IN SUCH A HOSTILE ENVIRONMENT. HE SMILED AND
TOLD HER THAT IN ALL THE GLOOM AND GREY WAS THE
MOST VIBRANT LIGHT AND COLOUR IN THE GRATITUDE
OF THOSE HE SHELTERED.

THE GODDESS PONDERED THIS FOR A MOMENT AND
THEN SHE BENT DOWN AND GAVE THE TREE A KISS. AS
SHE DID SO, A HUNDRED BEAUTIFUL, RED BERRIES BURST
FROM THE TREE'S BRANCHES, CAUSING THE LITTLE ONE
TO GIGGLE WITH DELIGHT.

"YOU SHALL BE KNOWN AS LUIS!" SHE TOLD HIM.
"DEFENDER OF THE WEAK AND PROTECTOR OF THE LOST
AND LONELY!"

AND FROM THAT DAY ONWARDS, LUIS GROWS A CROP OF
BRIGHT RED BERRIES TO DRAW EVEN MORE TRAVELLERS
TOWARDS HIM, SO THAT IN THE DARKNESS OF PLACES,
THERE IS FOOD, AND COLOUR, AND BIRDSONG.

The Mountain Ash or Rowan was traditionally deemed to be a highly protective tree and this is revealed in the saying "No evil shall pass the shadow of the Rowan".

The essence of Rowan contains this ability and much more as, in addition to the energy assertion it provides; it also gives the ability to halt negative reactions. Luis enables the discernment of whether you are being offered help or subjected to harmful intent.

The Rowan tree can survive in the most inhospitable places, breaking the murkiness with a vibrant display of red berries, attracting birds that shelter in its branches and fill the air with song.

This is another aspect of the Luis Essence—when things are at their darkest, when all is doom and gloom, hope has drained away and there seems to be no way out - Luis will fill the air with a beautiful song, light up the shadows with vibrant colour and shelter us from the worse effects of the environment.

Work on the Luis Essence was started in 2001 and took two years to evolve. Beginning with a very poorly 'dormant' Rowan that was nursed back to health over the period of a year.

The happier Rowan now needed to be set free and it was in a sacred grove on Bodmin Moor Grove that an ideal spot was found—almost as if it had been waiting for the little Rowan. So on a cold autumn night, the Rowan was released to a new life and there it still stands amongst its peers and the ancient ones who can pass on their wisdom.

Since that time, Rowan is another genus of our tree friends that is most popular with Celtic Reiki Masters. This, in turn, has created one of the richest and most diverse essences of Celtic Reiki that is available to us.

Whether connecting to the root essence of Luis or to the individual trees, we find so many loving and supportive elements to this aspect of energy that it is sometimes overwhelming in scope.

Physical: Boosts the immune system and helps with cold and flu symptoms. Helps to ease tea and sugar addictions.

Emotional/Mental: Mental clarity and discernment are major aspects of this essence, along with the ability to assert emotionally and mentally, for example, from the likes of depression, despair and loneliness; when all hope has disappeared. Also stimulates creativity.

Spiritual: Spiritual protection and awakening.

THE ORACLE OF LUIS

Luis reminds you that you are safe within the comforting waves of his essence. Traditionally used for protection, the Rowan is here to act as a guardian and keep you safe no matter what your current situation or circumstances. If you feel unsure of yourself, frightened or afraid, Rowan's ingression into your reading, signifies that he is here for you, keeping a watchful eye and ensuring that you can rest easy.

The Rowan or Mountain Ash can grow in the most inhospitable of places, lashed by the burning wind, ravaged by the rain and cold, starved from light and nutrients, the Rowan, produces vibrant red berries to feed the wildlife in his care. In doing so, he attracts songbirds, bring music and colour to the most barren and bleak landscapes.

If you feel that you life is bleak and dark, the Rowan shall bring you comfort, warmth and colour. The Luis essence will help you smile again, no matter what has happened, or how low you feel – he is here for you now.

If you are currently at a good place in your life, Rowan has come to offer kindness and giving, two other traits in his multifaceted range of qualities.

He also asked that you pass on a kindness to those you meet and to remember that a helping hand does not need to cost. Maybe you are the one who can spread the Luis essence to those who need it at this time.

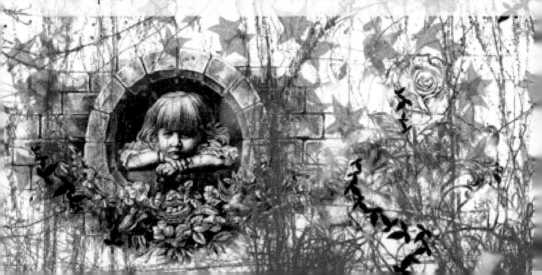

Fearn
Alder - F - [fi-een]

Several thousand years ago, a little bird came breathlessly from the south to land on a topmost branch of a young tree. Upon noticing the bird's breathless state, the tree enquired about what was wrong.

"Invaders are coming from the south to harm the human's that dwell in the forest!" cried the little bird.

"That is terrible!" replied the tree, "I must warn them before the invaders get here!"

"No! No!" whistled the bird, "Do not get involved in the affairs of human's, for once you are involved, you become a part of their folly!"

Ignoring the little bird's advice, the tree told a passing human of the impending invasion. The local became very upset and ran off to warn his clan, without even stopping to thank the tree for his kindness.

Soon a whole group of people from the clan returned to prepare for war and to make their weapons and defences, they chopped down all the trees in that part of the forest. As he waited his turn to be chopped down, the tree said to the little bird, "Please tell all of my kind what has happened here today and warn them never to share a secret or tell what must not be told!"

The little bird assured the tree that he would not rest until every tree of the Fearn tongue knew the value of secrets and hidden wisdom.

At the edge of a sacred grove in the northern mountains of Snowdonia, a huge lake lapped the steep slopes at the bottom of these mighty peaks and by the lake was a solitary Alder.

The tree was surrounded by stones that pulsed with energy, for the tree was a guardian of something very powerful. It was this tree that formed the basis for the Fearn Essence and it was created with the proviso that nothing physical be taken from the grove; no pebbles or sticks, no pinecones or hazelnuts.

This is the keeper of secrets and still to this day we do not know what the guardian of the grove was keeping in his care. Thus the Fearn Essence can be used on those who have the heavy spiritual 'burden' of secrets and the unknown – ancient and futuristic powers that they cannot share with others and thus are bound to silence.

It will also help those who are told the secrets of others and thus have a great power. It will help them to use their power wisely and be at ease with the responsibility they hold.

The Fearn Essence is also about remembrance and the passing of all things, it helps us to remember those we have lost and keep their memory alive within us. It also helps us to remember the things that we try to push aside, because we think they are too painful.

By embracing what we fear most, we can connect to the energy and then repattern it to something that gives us strength—by avoiding our past and suppressing it, we give it more power, so it haunts us. If we learn to remember our past from a new perspective and one that helps us to grow, we can also discover our greatest gifts and potential.

Another use for Fearn is that of recapturing the memories of our past lives and those of our ancestral line, helping us to remove any unwanted karma that we have at a vibrational level.

As we envelop ourselves in the lives that have gone before us, we can use the Celtic Reiki essences to treat those traumas and diseases that, extending forward in time from the past, hold us back in the here and now.

Physical: Issues of the lumber area, hips and pelvis. Joint pain, arthritis and rheumatism are all eased by the treatment with Fearn.

Emotional/Mental: Emotional force and strength of character, rather like the Duir Essence, yet more 'active' inasmuch as the Fearn Essence is more of a watchman than a gatekeeper. Thus, any situation that calls for a dynamic approach to assertiveness and action will benefit with this essence.

Spiritual: Higher task and a sense of mission.

THE ORACLE OF FEARN

The Alder tree says 'come on, keep going!'—for those who are carrying a spiritual burden, or who are facing a time of major challenge in their life. Fearn helps support you when you need her guidance and strength. She is particularly helpful of those who find themselves in a position of keeping secrets—because they are in a position of trust, or privilege, or because somebody has confessed something to them.

The keeper of Secrets is one with great power and much responsibility and this can be a role of great esteem and heavy weight. The Alder's presence is flowing from your reading and into the moments of your life, to ease your burden, keep you on your path and help you to keep your resolve – when you want her steadfast influence, simply call on her.

Fearn reminds us that to embrace what we fear most can be the most liberating and transformative action to take. No matter how frightening a situation may be, the fact that it provokes a fear response suggests that you need to take some action.

The Alder will assist you in taking that action, because whilst fear is there to help you, once you are alerted to its presence, it has served its purpose—fear that lingers, simply holds you back and keeps you prisoner – so break free from fear and move beyond it—to a world of courageous and definite action.

The Alder can represent a period of nostalgia and remembrance—thinking of those we have loved and lost, reminiscing about happy times spent with friends and family, or reliving an exciting event or adventure to rekindle your emotions now. Perhaps it is time to remove old challenges with your expanded perception and move on from traumatic memories using your mature perspective of now.

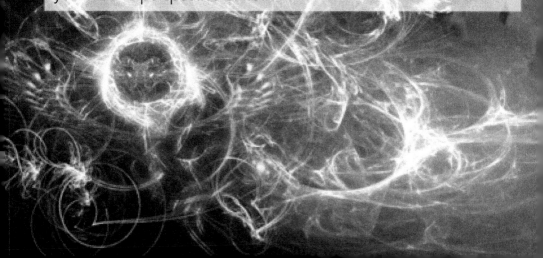

SAILLE
WILLOW - S - [SAL-YUR]

ONCE, THERE WAS SO MUCH PAIN IN THE WORLD OF HUMANS THAT THE TREES COULD STAND IT NO MORE AND DECIDED TO HELP THE PEOPLE OF THE WOODLAND REALM TO HEAL THEMSELVES. THE TREES HELD A MEETING BY WHISPERING ON THE WIND AND THROUGH THE SONG OF THE FOREST BIRDS; THEY SPOKE THROUGH THE GROUND AND IN THE GENTLE WAFT OF LEAF AND BRANCH. THIS MEETING WENT ON FOR SEVERAL MONTHS, WITHOUT ARRIVING AT ANY CONCLUSIONS.

SOME OF THE TREES SAID THAT THE HUMANS HELD SO MUCH OF THEIR PAIN INSIDE AND NEEDED TO RELEASE THEIR EMOTIONS. OTHER TREES SAID THAT PEOPLE WERE VERY FRAGILE AND BROKE TOO EASILY WHEN FACED WITH LIFE'S CHALLENGES. THEN THERE WERE THOSE WHO FELT THAT HUMANS WERE SO NAIVE TO THE WAYS OF THE WORLD THAT THEY WOULD BE BEST HELPED BY LARGE DOSES OF COMMON SENSE.

AS THE AUTUMN APPROACHED AND STILL WITH NO RESOLUTION TO THEIR DISCUSSIONS, THE TREES STARTED TO BELIEVE THAT PEOPLE NEEDED SO MUCH HELP THAT THEY WERE BEYOND HELP! THIS WAS UNTIL ONE GROUP OF TREES CAME UP WITH AN IDEA. SOME OF THEM WOULD WEEP INTO THE EARTH TO SHOW THE HUMANS HOW TO RELEASE THEIR PAIN AND TO SUPPORT THEIR CLEARING OF THE PAST. A FEW OF THE GROUP LEARNED HOW TO BREAK CLEANLY IN THE WIND, SO THAT THEIR DAMAGE WAS LIMITED AND REPAIR COULD BE CONDUCTED QUICKLY. AND THE REST BECAME MASTERS IN HEALING THE MOST COMMON ISSUES THAT FACED HUMANKIND.

THESE TREES; THE WEEPING, THE CRACK, AND THE COMMON, BECAME KNOWN AS SAILLE: HEALER OF THOSE IN PAIN AND GIVER OF WISDOM.

Saille is the Willow Tree and refers to the moon/lunar rhythms and as such has a very interesting nature. Firstly, the essence works in relation to the lunar cycle; therefore she is excellent at manifestation when the Moon is waxing (New to Full Moon) and treatment when the Moon is waning.

Next of all, the willow has many interesting qualities, not only in treating others and manifestation techniques, but also when working with other natural energy.

Willow eases pain of all kinds, physical, emotional, psychological and spiritual, she also works well on skin conditions, any issue to do with the hair and issues of the heart.

When used for fulfilment of wishes and dreams, Saille is best used in manifestations of the soul: to improve the ability to connect to higher levels, to work with guides, to help you clarify your life's work and discover your purpose. Saille is the manifestation tool for the spiritual that have travelled their path for a while and are ready for the next step. She will help you connect to work with ley lines and Stargates (Stone Circles) and connect you to the stars.

Willow was one of the first Celtic Reiki Essences, created with the help of a garden-bound Willow in London. She was an incredibly happy soul who enjoyed the sunlight and was very happy just 'being'.

One thing that stood out about this tree was her motherly nature, as she projected love to all the other flowers, plants and trees in the garden to make sure that they were all happy too. When the Willow was happy, all around her were happy, especially the flowers, growing under her branches; they appeared to be the happiest bunch one could wish to meet

Willows are often associated with grief—this is not due to the fact that they are unhappy, it is because they have long been located where there is much grief—so they can take it away…

A major development of the Saille Essence is the addition of 'Feather Willow', an ancient, ivy-covered willow in Cornwall. This tree is very interesting, not only for its wisdom, but also as it possesses neither male nor female qualities—it is androgynous, meaning that it is of a gender that we do not have in humankind, or the gender than can only be obtained by artificial means.

This means that Feather Willow can offer us a genderless perspective in issues of gender, such as communication difficulties between men and women, or problems with gender identity. For those who identify with a gender that is different to their birth gender or those who were born hermaphrodite, Saille works in creating understanding and truly positive identity.

Thus Saille is not about 'coming to terms with' or 'accepting' one's gender identity or gender issues – it is about revelation and true comprehension of our very individual and personal gender: creating equality and self-esteem within the individual that will be reflected outwards.

The trees do not have sexual politics – they just are who they are and do what they do without judgement of others or themselves. These qualities can also be instilled, not only in people who have difficulty with their own gender or sexual identity, but in those who hate others because of gender or sexual preference.

Sexuality and gender-related issues affect us on physical, emotional and psychological levels but have no place in true spirituality, so cannot affect us there. However, as we grow up and develop, the second-hand limiting, dogmatic and prejudicial beliefs of our society and those individuals hungry for power, domination and control through blame, affect us and can create spiritual dilemmas.

Saille can help us to view those of different gender and sexual identity as equals, with equal rights – this means that we accept all genders and sexualities within ourselves, so that we embrace our own sexual/gender identity completely.

Two other layers of the Saille Essence are derived from Willow trees that have been near death and yet recovered – one is a weeping willow, the other a corkscrew willow. Both of these trees nearly died, the corkscrew through lack of water and the weeping willow as it had been placed into a dormant state and packaged for sale in a convenience store. It never truly recovered from this, however the rootstock started to grow again, enabling the growth of a new tree to start.

Both of these small, yet beautiful individuals

encompass the qualities of the original Saille Essence, yet here the meaning of survival after death and spiritual rebirth are apparent when we realise we can even overcome physical death to live on and whilst there is the smallest flicker of hope, we can make it through the pain.

Physical: Pain, such as headache and muscular ache/pain. Skin conditions, hair loss, dandruff, etc. Heartburn, pain in the chest and heart. Physical illness caused by deep-rooted trauma.

Emotional/Mental: Emotional and Mental anguish. Trauma of all kinds. To soothe and calm the nerves and release bitterness/resentment from the heart area. Can also be used to make somebody laugh!

Spiritual: Use in powerful manifestations such as astral travel, vibrational bi-location, avatar qualities, ancient energy and communications, multidimensional work.

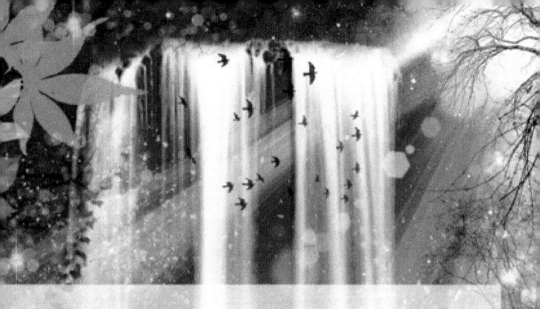

The Oracle of Saille

The Willow is one of the most powerful and transformative essences of Celtic Reiki and if she is visiting you at a time of pain, trauma or ill-health, it will not last long, for Saille is here to alleviate your hurt.

The motherly willow bends towards you, wraps you up, safe and warm in her branches and relieves all your pain and grief; she washes away any emotion that causes you hurt and leaves you to sleep in a serene state of absolute bliss.

The willow also helps to clarify issues of gender and sexuality – removing limiting beliefs that have been instilled by others and helping you to be more comfortable with your gender and sexual nature.

If you have been facing challenges that are connected these, it is not simply a case of acceptance or 'coming to terms with'—it is about pride and absolute love of yourself, no matter of your sex or sexual identity.

Saille whispers of mysteries, hidden power and ancient mystical arts. She helps you uncover deceit and arm yourself with knowledge. She gives insight into unspoken wisdom that can help you in your current situation, and she invites you to listen to the messages and see the signs that are all around you now.

Willow knows answers that most cannot know and she is willing to let you in on the secret!

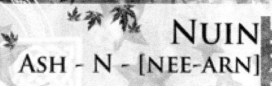

NUIN
ASH - N - [NEE-ARN]

DURING THE AGE.OF AN ANCIENT AND TERRIBLE WAR, THERE LIVED A WISE TREE WHO COMMANDED ALL OTHER TREES. HE WAS KNOWN AS NUIN AND HE WAS A FAIR AND POWERFUL TREE KING, WHO WAS VERY SAD TO SEE THE HUMANS KILLING EACH OTHER AND DESTROYING THE BEAUTY OF THE EARTH.

ONE DAY A COMMANDER OF ONE OF THE ARMIES CAME TO THE KING NUIN AND TOLD HIM THAT THE OPPOSING ARMY WERE BURNING DOWN THE GREAT FORESTS OF THE EAST AND WOULD HE PLEASE HELP THE COMMANDER TO STOP THIS AWFUL DESTRUCTION. EAGER TO HELP PUT AN END TO THE WAR, NUIN SAID THAT HE WOULD HELP THE COMMANDER.

THE TREE KING LISTENED AS THE COMMANDER SAID THAT IF HE HAD NUIN'S PERMISSION TO CHOP DOWN A FEW T REES, HE COULD CREATE MORE POWERFUL WEAPONS AND DEFEAT THE ARMY TO THE EAST. AT THIS TIME, TREES COULD NOT BE CHOPPED DOWN WITHOUT THE TREE KING'S PERMISSION AND ANYBODY WHO TRIED WOULD HAVE NOTHING BUT A BROKEN AXE AND BLUNTED SAW.

THE COMMANDER REQUESTED THAT NUIN WRITE DOWN HIS PERMISSION TO CHOP DOWN OTHER TREES TO HELP STOP THE WAR. NUIN WAS HESITANT AT FIRST, BUT KNEW THAT SOMETHING MUST BE DONE, SO USED SOME OF HIS BARK AND SAP TO WRITE A REQUEST THAT COULD BE SHOWN TO THE TREES. THE COMMANDER TOOK THIS AWAY WITH HIM AND PROMPTLY BUILT HIS WEAPONS AND WON THE WAR.

HOWEVER, EVEN WHEN PEACE PREVAILED, THE COMMANDER AND HIS KIN USED NUIN'S WRITTEN PERMISSION TO CLEAR HUGE AREAS OF FOREST, EVEN THOUGH THE KING NOW PROTESTED. SO, FROM THAT DAY FORTH, THE NUIN REMINDS US NEVER TO WRITE DOWN WHAT NEEDS TO CHANGE AT SOME FUTURE DATE.

Since the creation of Celtic Reiki, several Ash trees have contributed to the Nuin Essence from their own, unique perspective. One of the common themes with Ash is that, compared with the likes of Quert, Tinne or Saille, Nuin tends to lean more to the intellectual or cerebral aspects of perspective.

Yet, unlike the other trees of knowledge, Nuin works in a very different way to Phagos, who enthuses knowledge like a child who has learnt something new and cannot wait to tell the world, or Huathe, who offers little chunks of information a piece at a time.

Even Coll, the tree of knowledge, gathers her wisdom through 'gossiping' and hearsay – she is like the housekeeper who sees all and knows all the goings-on of the house, yet in the case of Hazel, she tells all – to everybody who will listen!

Nuin prefers to infer knowledge through example, creating action or reaction to his essence that enables you to see the essence of the lesson played out before you. He is logical and practical, yet extremely benevolent and just a touch humorous in his style. If trees had jobs, he would be the college professor who is always one-step ahead of his students and has the ability to make you feel very big or very small.

Physical: Balancing between left and right body. Health issues that affect one side of the body more than the other, or that change from one side to the other.

Emotional/Mental: Transmission of knowledge and the gathering of wisdom. Balance of mind and emotions.

Spiritual: The sacred nature of spiritual knowledge. Fluidity of perspective and the oral traditions of spirit wisdom. Expansion and growth

THE MESSAGE OF NUIN

I am a path that grows straight ahead, yet when I develop branches, they form at the same place and stretch out in opposite directions. Thus, I offer a choice—to call upon our spiritual and higher aspects, to move towards the practical and logical path, or to continue on the path of balance. The answer may be different on each occasion, but all paths will eventually lead to the light.

I teach the inner and the outer, the very large in the very small – I am a paradox and an understanding that can only be felt and known, rather than understood.

My essence can be called upon whenever you are dealing with many small issues or in times of huge change. Where you encounter contrast and opposition, you may call upon me for guidance.

I also help on all levels, when dealing with the large and the small, such as the small in-growing toenail that affects the way you posture your entire body or the tiny worry that is blown out of proportion.

I can help you on the path to enlightenment when the tiniest of blockages has completely halted your progress and I am always ready to help you work through the straw that breaks the camel's back!

Traditionally used as the connection during the beginning of a treatment or Orientation, I initiate the end – for beginnings are always ending.

I represent both the start of the treatment and the finish of dis-ease, the commencement of a new path towards the use of Celtic Reiki Essences and the ending of old struggles and beliefs. My season is the first month of spring and while I represent the creation of new hopes and dreams for the coming year, I also encompass an end to the harsh months of winter.

Whenever you work with my perspective, observe what is not seen, what is not known and whilst you may not be able to truly grasp the hidden dynamics of my perspective, be aware that in everything there is opposition and balance.

THE ORACLE OF NUIN

The Ash expands the reach of his branches towards you, to lift you upwards and, as you soar towards the sky, he speaks in the hushed tones of the wind. He tells us of knowledge, but not the written information that all can see—he speaks of tradition, carried down for generations and of that, whispered to us from places in time that we have not seen—yet—for Nuin is connected to future as well as the past.

Who you will become, already exists at some point in time – and whilst you have many choices to make between here and there, the essence of Nuin is like a map that will help you find your way to the most perfect future you could ever desire. For as your future self calls back through time, offering advice, giving instructions and showing you the way forward, the Ash tree is listening!

Ash is also a great balancer – of left and right, logic and emotion, the great and the small. He assists with problem-solving; of focussing when you are 'all over the place' or of awareness when you are too honed on a particular aspect of a challenge.

He helps with difficult or even impossible decisions, creating equilibrium between the head and heart. He offers the smallest of details in the greatest of plans and the bigger-picture when all you see is nuts and bolts.

The Nuin essence is humorous and invites you to laugh and play and be happy. If you have little reason to smile or have fun, the Ash will remind you of what it is to be a child and to find excitement in even the most restrictive and limiting of circumstance. It is time to unleash your imagination, to think creativity and playfully and most of all to laugh loudly and clearly!

HUATHE
HAWTHORN - H - [HOO-ARTH]

AROUND THE TIME WHEN THE REALMS OF HUMANS AND TREES FIRST CAME TO MEET, A LITTLE TREE SPROUTED FROM THE GROUND, JOYOUS AND EXCITED THAT HE WOULD GET TO MEET SO MANY NEW FRIENDS, BOTH TREE AND HUMAN. THE TINY FELLOW WAS BORN WITH THE MOST FEARSOME THORNS, HOWEVER, AND PEOPLE SOON LEARNED NOT TO GO NEAR HIM FOR FEAR OF BEING CUT, PRICKED OR SLICED!

GRADUALLY FEWER PEOPLE DWELT NEAR THE LITTLE TREE AND AS HE GREW INTO ADULTHOOD, HE BECAME VERY LONELY. SO, WHEN A WEARY TRAVELLER STOPPED TO REST NEARBY ON A HOT SUMMER'S DAY, THE PRICKLY TREE MADE SURE HE KEPT VERY STILL FOR FEAR OF SCARING THE MAN AWAY.

"OH!" CRIED THE MAN, "I WISH I HAD SOME WATER AND FOOD TO HELP ME ON MY JOURNEY!"

NO SOONER HAD THE MAN ASKED FOR THESE, THAN A POUCH OF WATER AND A LOAF OF BREAD FELL AT HIS FEET. THE MAN, SPUN AROUND, LOOKING FOR THE ONE WHO HAD GIVEN HIM THE FOOD.

"WHO HAS DONE THIS?" ASKED THE MAN, CALLING TO THE WIND AND THE SKY.

"IT WAS I!" WHISPERED THE TREE, FOR HE WAS OF THE HUATHE CLAN AND THEY POSSESSED THE POWERS OF MAGIC AND MANIFESTATION.

"WHATEVER CAN I DO TO REPLAY THIS KINDNESS?" ASKED THE TRAVELLER, WALKING UP TO THE TREE.

"PLEASE TIE A PIECE OF YOUR CLOTHING AROUND MY THORNS TO STOP ME FROM HURTING THOSE WHO PASS." THE LITTLE HUATHE REPLIED.

THE TRAVELLER TORE SOME OF THE FABRIC FROM HIS SHIRT AND TIED IT INTO A KNOW AROUND ONE OF THE TREE BRANCHES. AS HE DID THIS, THE MAN AND TREE TALKED AND SHARED THEIR STORIES. AFTERWARDS, THE MAN DRANK SOME WATER AND ATE BREAD, WHILST THEY CONTINUED TO TALK WELL INTO THE NIGHT.

THE FOLLOWING MORNING, THE TRAVELLER SET OFF ON HIS VOYAGE ONCE AGAIN. ON THE WAY, HE MET MANY FOLK AND HE TOLD THEM WHAT HAD HAPPENED AND IT WAS NOT LONG BEFORE PEOPLE CAME FROM FAR AND WIDE TO OFFER CLOTHING TO HUATHE IN THE HOPE HE MIGHT GRANT THEIR WISHES ALSO.

Huathe is of the Hawthorn and his essence represents the force of cleansing and preparation. The clearing of thoughts, as distinct from physical actions. He is an excellent forerunner to the Beith essence; he clears the mind of negative thoughts and mental confusion, offering clarity. He gives patience and offers stillness and the ability to wait until the right time comes.

Can be used in conjunction with Ailim to calm and create a clear picture of the way ahead. Sometimes the way ahead can be obscured by too many thoughts; this will clear those thoughts, allowing Ailim to show the horizon.

Another use for the Hawthorn essence is in conception of life. It can be used to help increase fertility during the conception of a child, during the pregnancy and at the actual birth. Huathe will help smooth the process and create plain sailing for both mother and baby. The reverse is also appropriate, as this essence will help women through the menopause, lessening the harshest of the side effects.

Hawthorn is not the easiest of species to work with during the harvest process and has taken his fair share of blood (which surprisingly is the way of Huathe). There is often a price to be paid, but the rewards are great! Huathe is unlike any other species of tree; he is abrupt, to the point, acerbic and can be fickle – yet his wisdom and ability is second to none. He offers knowledge and magic from a very different perspective. In times of real need, this can be exactly what we need to get us through.

Hawthorne's ability to cleanse and prepare the way can often be misinterpreted as carelessness or may seem hurtful in its apparent lack of compassion, but Huathe does care – he just shows it in a very different way to other trees! Huathe enables us to realise that others do not appreciate us if we give ourselves freely – and when we give ourselves freely we assert to other levels of our being that we are not worth much. There must always be an exchange: a trade of information or of idea. To always give selflessly creates imbalance and that is never healthy.

Individuals in the Huathe Essence include the 'Old Hawthorne of Time' who gives us a very tree-oriented view of space and time and is very helpful to those who cannot grasp practical or physical concepts such as space (finding their way around) and time (can never get anywhere on time).

Seeing an alternative perspective, albeit energetically, can really help us to come to terms with physical concepts that we usually only see from a human or society-based viewpoint. There are many other ways of perceiving our world and not all of these take human form!

Another of the Huathe perspective is 'Clooty Hawthorne'. Clooties were small pieces of cloth that were traditionally knotted around the branches of the Hawthorne tree when a person wanted to make a wish for something.

Therefore, Clooty Hawthorne is an excellent choice when conducting a manifestation treatment or making a wish. Shift to his perspective and he will help you to make your dreams come true – remember that there may be a price to be paid. This may take the form of losing some money/an object or maybe a small cut or bruise – you can always pre-empt this by returning a favour to Hawthorne through your own freewill and volition.

Physical: Can be used in conjunction with IVF. Pregnancy and Childbirth. Menopause. Works on the circulatory system and reduces blood pressure.

Emotional/Mental: Can help in matters of the heart: in both healing and releasing relationships. Will help to save a love that is dying – providing this is for the highest good. Can help those wishing to manifest a loving relationship or who wish to be parents.

Spiritual: Can help to nurture unconditional, spiritual love for all things.

THE ORACLE OF HUATHE

Tie a Clooty to the branches of a Hawthorn and he will offer you gifts a plenty, for Huathe has the ability to grant wishes and fill your life with the energy of abundance! Yet, to achieve your heart's desire there are three steps to take—these steps correspond with the positioning of the Huathe essence in your reading and thus, here the past, present and future, represent, conception, growth, and completion.

The conception stage is a time for clearing the past away and making ready with new ideas, fresh plans and preparation for what you want to achieve.

This may also favour the conception of a child, the success of a first date, new friendships and relationships, or the achievement of original solutions and ideas. Whatever the specifics of your situation, the Hawthorn says that it is time to prepare, wipe clean, and aim yourself in the right direction.

The growth aspect of Huathe is of energising and building on what has gone before. Using the foundations you have already set in place, to construct something wonderful in readiness for what you will achieve.

This may also relate to maintaining your health and fitness, learning and growing your knowledge, nurturing friendships and loving relationships, or building in some way – energy, vibrancy and strength.

Finally the completion vibrations of Hawthorn simply say—clear your mind and relax, for all your effort and past action is about to become achievement. It is a time for success and achievement—your Clooty desire is about to arrive!

DUIR
OAK - D - [DOO-R]

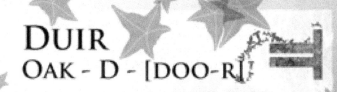

TREES, ON THE WHOLE, ARE WISE CREATURES.

THIS WAS NOT ALWAYS THE CASE WHEN IT CAME TO THEIR INTERACTIONS WITH HUMANS. TREES ONCE TREATED HUMANS WITH THE SAME TRUST AND OPENNESS THAT THEY HAVE FOR EACH OTHER. YET, THEIR DEALINGS WITH HUMANS SOON TAUGHT THEM CAUTION AND OVER TIME THIS BECAME A DEEP MISTRUST, ESPECIALLY FOR THOSE THAT HAVE BEEN TREATED BADLY BY PEOPLE.

SUCH AS THE FIRST TREE OF THE DUIR PERSPECTIVE, WHO WAS TRICKED INTO HOLDING OPEN A MAGICAL PORTAL FOR A DEVIOUS MAGICIAN. THE STRENGTH OF THE DUIR TREE WAS RENOWNED THROUGHOUT THE REALMS OF ALL LIVING THINGS AND SO WHEN ASKED TO TEST HIS PHYSICAL AND SPIRITUAL POTENCY BY HOLDING THE PORTAL HIGH AND KEEPING IT OPEN, THE FIRST DUIR ACCEPTED READILY. IT WAS ONLY LATER THAT HE REALISED HE HAD BEEN DECEIVED AND HE AND HIS KIND WAS DESTINED TO HOLD THE PORTAL OPEN UNTIL THE END OF TIME.

NOWADAYS, THE DUIR CLAN STILL HOLD OPEN MAGICAL GATEWAYS AND PORTALS. HOWEVER THEY ARE NOT AS EASY TO DISTRACT AND TEND TO AVOID CONTACT WITH HUMANS, UNTIL THEY PROVE THEIR TRUSTWORTHINESS!

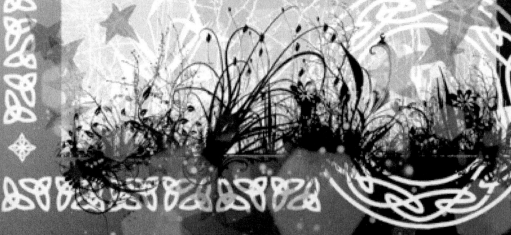

Duir is of the Oak Tree and represents the month of May, the last month of spring and the end of the beginning. Duir is an excellent perspective to align with near the completion of the first stages in a project. As the foundations of our work are complete, Duir will smooth over any rough edges and tie up any loose ends. Thus, he will help the transition to the next stage of a journey and is wonderful just before a full Moon.

Duir is the opener of doors and gateways. He lends those who have connected a great strength and knowledge of the mysteries contained in the universe. He protects and keeps the practitioner and client safe from any contraction during the treatment or practice.

The initial creation of Duir happened whilst conducting a treatment to an old Oak located in St James' Park, London. This mighty individual was very strong willed, but very benevolent towards his human visitors, feeling a great need to shelter people under his branches!

Oak trees containing Mistletoe were seen as the most sacred and honoured of trees by the Celts—there is something about the synthesis of Oak and Mistletoe that cannot be attained from any other perspective.

Physical: Back Pain, Diarrhoea, Food Poisoning and Fungal Infection. Addiction to Tea/Coffee.

Emotional/Mental: Lack of inner strength, weak and tossed about by life. Exceptional results to be found in those who are unable to put words or thoughts into action. People who hide the truth from others and themselves. Fear. Darkness.

Spiritual: Works well in manifestation and bringing the spiritual or energetic into physical reality. Offers a spiritual truth to the user and the receiver of the essence.

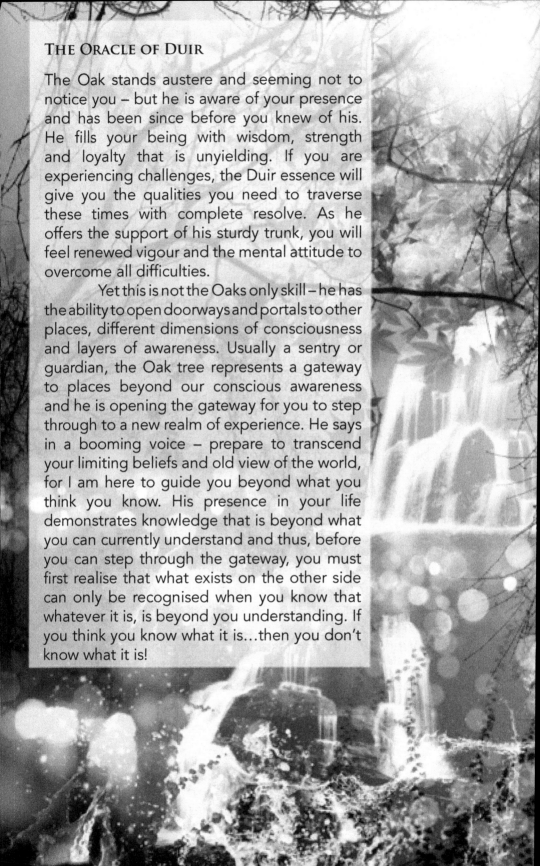

THE ORACLE OF DUIR

The Oak stands austere and seeming not to notice you – but he is aware of your presence and has been since before you knew of his. He fills your being with wisdom, strength and loyalty that is unyielding. If you are experiencing challenges, the Duir essence will give you the qualities you need to traverse these times with complete resolve. As he offers the support of his sturdy trunk, you will feel renewed vigour and the mental attitude to overcome all difficulties.

Yet this is not the Oaks only skill – he has the ability to open doorways and portals to other places, different dimensions of consciousness and layers of awareness. Usually a sentry or guardian, the Oak tree represents a gateway to places beyond our conscious awareness and he is opening the gateway for you to step through to a new realm of experience. He says in a booming voice – prepare to transcend your limiting beliefs and old view of the world, for I am here to guide you beyond what you think you know. His presence in your life demonstrates knowledge that is beyond what you can currently understand and thus, before you can step through the gateway, you must first realise that what exists on the other side can only be recognised when you know that whatever it is, is beyond you understanding. If you think you know what it is…then you don't know what it is!

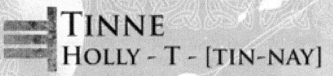

Tinne
Holly - T - [TIN-NAY]

The Once was a tree who wanted to be a mother so badly that she gave her seeds to all that passed in the hope they would plant them for her in fertile ground. However, the sweet and juicy berries in which her seeds were contained, became so sought after that they were often taken without a thought for the trees wishes.

So, she grow sharp ridges on her leaves to protect her berries from those who were unwilling to help her in return. It was no long, though, before crafty thieves learnt how to take her berries without being caught by her leaves.

Tired from producing so many berries, the tree asked the Lord Cernunnos for help. He replied by making the tree's berries poisonous to all, except those who plant her seed as promised. In return the tree must be a mother to all who ask for her help and nurture. Thus, she became known as Tinne, the Universal mother and protector of all those in need.

The Holly is the protector of the Ogham. Unlike Luis, which guards from contractive reactions to energy and influences, Tinne empowers an individual, enabling them to fight their own battles. The increased vigour and resilience produced by the Tinne Essence allows people to assert themselves, especially when engaged in struggle where balance is required along with the need to 'keep it together'.

Traditionally seen as masculine or father energy, Holly can also be regarded as the maternal nurturer for, within the hard exterior of those spiny leaves, is a soft heart and over-powering love that is given completely unconditionally.

Hence, Tinne, acting as both father and mother, female and male, can show us an all-encompassing love that shows us how to love ourselves in a completely balanced way and from all perspectives.

The wisdom of Holly is unquestionable, automatically bringing to the light an answer to the most complex life question. There is often, however, a sacrifice to be made with Tinne Essence, as it can be the case that, to find an answer, you may need to give something up. It is only afterwards that you realise you never needed it.

Physical: Pain relief. Speeds healing of broken bones. Sexual disease, or dysfunction.

Emotional/Mental: Calming, soothing and stress releasing. Holly can raise a fighting spirit or show the need for reconciliation or peace. Especially beneficial with deep-rooted anger, hate, jealousy and desire for revenge. Holly can help everybody to understand their sexuality, work with gender issues and integrate inner male/female aspects of their psyche.

Spiritual: Can provide sudden inspiration and intuitive knowledge. Gives an individual the ability to 'pluck answers out of the air'.

THE ORACLE OF TINNE

The Mother, the protector, the comforter and the Queen – she is Tinne, the most regal and beautiful. She symbolises the power of all her kind; fierce and deadly, noble and proud—she stands aloft and purveys her dominion. She gazes upon you with an air of absolute austerity and says…You need a cuddle, little one!

For she is the mother—she is bedtime stories and hot cocoa, she is warm snuggles and a soft-voice song. She wraps her arms around you and you feel completely loved and cherished. For Tinne is the essence of motherhood and the matriarch.

Within her world, her realm, you will always be safe and loved. She will protect and guide, sometimes she will challenge and expect more than you feel yourself capable of, however, she never stops loving and caring for her children.

And remember—when you are wrapped in this Tinne essence, there is no sense of the outside world—of what lies beyond these soft, comforting waves of energy. Outside, she is the most fearsome defender and is working with all her might and fury to stave off your troubles and fears and she will never fail. So relax, be warm and sip your hot chocolate, for you are loved and always shall be loved.

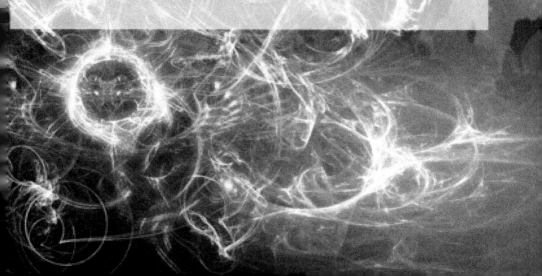

Coll
Hazel - C - [CULL]

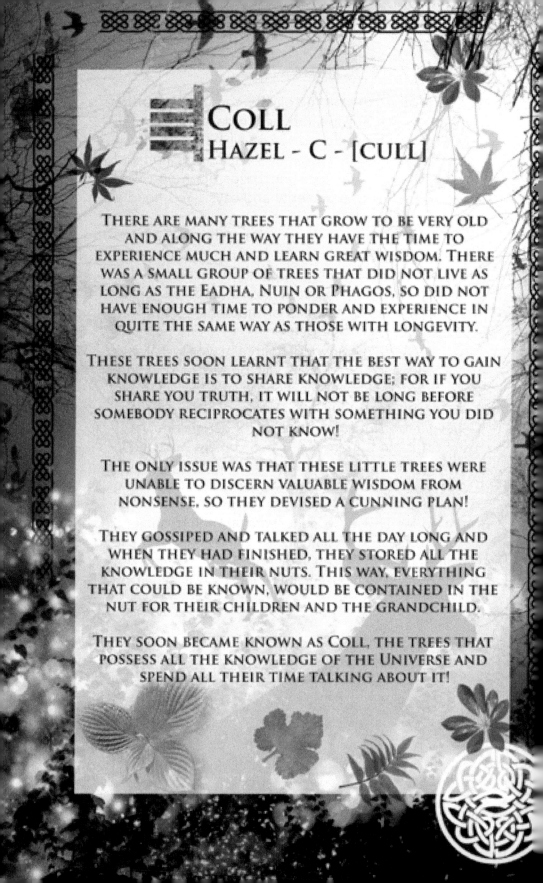

There are many trees that grow to be very old and along the way they have the time to experience much and learn great wisdom. There was a small group of trees that did not live as long as the Eadha, Nuin or Phagos, so did not have enough time to ponder and experience in quite the same way as those with longevity.

These trees soon learnt that the best way to gain knowledge is to share knowledge; for if you share you truth, it will not be long before somebody reciprocates with something you did not know!

The only issue was that these little trees were unable to discern valuable wisdom from nonsense, so they devised a cunning plan!

They gossiped and talked all the day long and when they had finished, they stored all the knowledge in their nuts. This way, everything that could be known, would be contained in the nut for their children and the grandchild.

They soon became known as Coll, the trees that possess all the knowledge of the Universe and spend all their time talking about it!

Coll is the Hazel, one of the most revered and valued trees in the age of the Celts. It was called the 'Tree of Knowledge' and the centre of all knowledge was believed to be contained in the Hazelnut, a very potent symbol for the Celts. The wood from the Hazel is said to have mystical powers and has long been sought after by those of the Wiccan faith for use in wands and staffs.

The Coll essence reflects this in her ability to enhance personal knowledge and awareness and, when used in a treatment, she can help to increase awareness in all aspects of the self. For example: the Coll perspective can put a person in touch with their body so that they will know what foods they need, how much physical activity they should partake in, what is harming their body, etc.

The Coll Essence can also put people in touch with other parts of themselves, such as their emotions, their higher self, their true self, etc.

The Hazel was also seen as the 'Emblem of Healing' and is therefore very therapeutic when used as a general 'tonic'. She will help increase your wisdom and inspiration in consultation environments and generally sensitise your intuitive abilities during a treatment.

Coll can also increase the potency of all other essences, especially of Oir and the two work very well together. Another aspect of the Hazel Essence is that of the nut, which is also a part of the Essence of Coll.

What we sometimes do not understand about Hazels is how they get their information – of course the answer exists with the fact that the Hazels are the world's biggest gossips!

Hazel's art for hearsay is second to none as she chatters away constantly. The Hazel is never malicious or cruel in what she says, always laughing and keeping her dignity, but she has found that the best way to know all is to tell all!

The Coll Essence reflects this quality, as it offers us knowledge yet it is the wisdom of hearsay. In our factual world, we tend to trust books more than the Internet. If we see facts in an encyclopaedia, they are truer than the words of somebody we meet on the street and, if it is on the television - well, that is more factual than anything else!

However we tend to attract in the information that we

need at the time it is most relevant so, whether it is spoken or written in a book—the important thing is that it resonates.

It is better to believe something that fits perfectly with you and makes you happy, than to replace your beliefs with a fact that gives you no comfort and offers nothing but darkness – this is not deceiving oneself, for who actually has the right to say something is true and something is false? Everything, absolutely everything is perspective and hearsay, even science.

Coll will tell you exactly what you need to know, when you need to know it – so trust her. She may seem like a giggly schoolgirl on the surface, but she is a wise and loving woman, capable of the most profound wisdom and the most resonant knowledge.

Physical: Very good at enabling a person to look after their body better. Boost physical healing. Cigarette and Alcohol additions.

Emotional/Mental: Helps to calm and empower a person emotionally. Can lead a person to their life path and to recognise their positive and negative traits. Wisdom.

Spiritual: Increases spiritual knowledge and soul's journey. Good for use in self-treatment for all Energy Therapists.

THE ORACLE OF COLL

Can you hear a giggling? A soft, clandestine whisper? There is intrigue afoot and the Hazel Trees are right in the centre of it. The Essence of Coll in your reading may tell of scandal or gossiping. Maybe tongues are wagging and you don't know who to trust.

Whispers can be comforting, they can also be cruel, for once they are offered to the breeze, who knows where they will end up. The best way to end gossip is to simply walk away—detach yourself from it, for whilst it may have momentum while you are a part of it, as soon as you remove yourself, it has nothing to feed upon and will die.

The Hazel offers you a nut—a hazelnut—it contains all the knowledge in the world—attained, not through books or academia, but through word of mouth, through experience, through sharing of perspective.

There is wisdom in the old wives tale and the folklore, the fable and the allegory. The Coll essence is of all these things. She drops the most profound understanding you will ever know into your lap, giggles and runs away, leaving you wide eyed and wonderful.

Her presence in a reading, not only reflects power and insight into the other essences here, but also offers you a tonic – healing waves of energy that create vibrancy and a sense of wellbeing.

As you walk on from her presence, you'll feel a bounce in your step and a frolic in your heart as you skip onwards with vigour and a sense of awareness.

QUERT
APPLE - Q - [KWERT]

BEAUTY AND LOVE ARE GIFTS...

...THE TREES LONG TO EXPERIENCE AND NONE MORE SO
THAN THOSE OF THE QUERT FAMILY. THE FIRST OF
THEIR KIND WAS SO DESPERATE TO EXPERIENCE THESE
FLEETING AND MOST VALUABLE OF TREASURES THAT
SHE GREW THE JUICIEST, SWEETEST AND PLUMPEST
FRUIT IN THE WHOLE OF THE WOODLAND REALM.

HER FRUIT BECAME SO RENOWN FOR ITS TASTE THAT
PEOPLE WOULD COME FROM ALL OVER THE REALMS TO
SAVOUR THEM. EVENTUALLY, THOSE WHO CAME,
WOULD MEET, TALK AND FORM RELATIONSHIPS UNDER
HER BRANCHES, SO SHE WAS ABLE TO SEE ALL THE LOVE
AND BEAUTY SHE COULD EVER WISH FOR.

IT WAS NOT LONG BEFORE THE MESSAGE OF HER KIND
BECAME THAT OF GIVING FIRST, WITHOUT THE HOPE
OF RECEIVING IN RETURN. FOR WHEN YOU CREATE
FLOW BY GIVING, IT IS UNIVERSAL LORE THAT YOU MUST
ALSO RECEIVE!

Quert is the perspective of love and beauty that can be used wherever there is a lack of both, whether this is a true lack or a perceived one. When treating those who feel unloved or who cannot see the beauty within them, Quert will fill their world with a harmony, peace and joy that is formed from the vibrant and essential energy of love and beauty.

Quert raises a person's self-esteem and enhances a well-rounded and realistic love of oneself, particularly useful in times of darkness or when feeling unappreciated by those around you.

The essence is that of gratitude and faith—of trusting in the processes of life and the wonder of the Universe and of being thankful for all that life has to offer. Especially valuable when we are focused on the three-dimensional aspects of physical life and forget about the amazing gifts we receive each day but often overlook.

Physically, Quert works on the gastric system and the chest—excellent for any disease surrounding the heart or solar plexus chakras. It is therefore wonderful when used on asthma, bronchitis, pneumonia or upper digestive complaints, etc. Quert is an excellent cleanser and can help to clean the gut and the blood and is excellent when combating the symptoms of high-cholesterol.

The apple tree perspective also works well on mental and spiritual levels, helping a person to find and fulfil their destiny, to assist in the meeting of a soulmate or increase the love and passion within an ailing relationship. It also helps a person retain their generosity in times when things are tight and one might not feel like giving. Quert combines well with Luis and Ruis.

This particular essence was originally harvested in the Cornish grove that has played such an integral part in the development of Celtic Reiki. A single crab apple tree stands in the Grove – it is right by the main road passing through this sacred place and yet is unseen and often missed by those passing. This friendly and loving individual completes the 'Sacred Tree' essences of the Celts and enhances the Koad Essence also.

Physical: Chest and stomach issues. General cleansing qualities, especially of the colon and the blood.

Emotional/Mental: Beauty and love, especially Universal love or compassion. Quert helps us transition into the 'I Care' and 'Universal Care' stages of life, transcending selfishness and egocentric views of the world, in favour of a giving viewpoint.

Spiritual: Spiritual expansion and compassion. Powerful manifestation and energy-magic abilities.

THE ORACLE OF QUERT

The Apple Tree speaks to you of love—it's in the air and everywhere you look! Around you, everywhere you go and in all you meet. Remember the first throws of love, of meeting and falling and relishing every breath, every flower, every word. Colours more colourful, sounds are sweeter, you can't think of anything else and feel fit to burst with happiness.

Well this is the message the Quert essence brings to you. She swans in on a pink, fluffy cloud of energy, waves her magic wand and everything in a boring, drab world becomes tinted with rainbow sparkles and the sweet scent of apple blossom.

As you may guess, relationships are highlighted by the Quert essence—new love affairs, a deepening of existing love or the creation of lasting, loving friendships. There is an innate beauty in everything the Apple Tree touches with her influence—she wraps herself around your life and suddenly it will be giggling under the bed covers at 4am, long walks in the park, log fires after getting caught in the rain and candle-lit dinners for two. It is day trips to Paris and weekends away. It is afternoons chatting and nights on the town.

Love, is about to enter your life—completely, utterly, totally in all its many-splendored-thing-ness. So grab an apple, hold on tight to the nearest trunk and prepare to wring every last drop of joy from the moments offered, saturating your life with happy memories and overwhelming love.

Muin

Blackberry|Vine - M - [MHOOWN]

There once was a tree that had been given so much from her parents that she became very spoilt. Each day, her demands would become more and more outlandish, from twinkly-sparkles to decorate each of her branches, to pillywiggin juice to moisturise her leaves.

Eventually her parents died and the little tree was left alone to find her own twinkly-sparkles and squeeze pillywiggins with her own twigs!

One day, a woodland deity, who shall remain anonymous for legal reasons, was passing dressed in her finest pillywiggin costume. The little tree spied her flitting past and grabbed her by the ankles.

"You'll make a beautiful twinkly-sparkle for one of my twigs!" Exclaimed the tree, "But not before I've squeezed you completely dry of your juice!"

"You really are rather yucky!" Cried the woodland deity who in that moment transformed to her usual appearance. "For being so rude and for bullying your fellow woodland dwellers, I hereby decree that you shall live this day forth as an ugly, spiky bush that will frighten away all who look upon you!"

All at once, the tree became gnarled and twisted, growing large, hooked spikes that tore the flesh of all who passed by.

Soon nobody ventured near the little bush and she became very lonely. For many years she reflected on her behaviour towards others and began to weep with remorse. With every tear that she cried luscious, sweet berry appeared on her branches and it was not long before the birds and other creatures came to eat the berries and offer the bush company in return.

Thus, the Muin Essence came to be and the bramble become one of the most loved of the woodland, even though she still has a bit of a reputation for being a bit prickly!

Muin encompasses the vines, and in the case of the Celtic Reiki Muin Essence the Bramble, or Blackberry. This prickly, somewhat intimidating plant is one of the most prolific and hardy creatures in England, found commonly amongst the hedgerows that border our roads and lanes.

This can be somewhat troublesome for the unwary hiker, yet they offer an abundant source of food for birds, animals and us blackberry lovers come September – the month of Muin.

Muin is balance and diplomacy, for it is equally defensive and enticing, for it offers a nasty cut to those who mistreat it, but riches to those who act with care in its presence. The essence of Muin inherits this trait and gives us a range of perception unlike any other. This particular aspect of energy is used without intent and just projected at times you intuit during treatments, self-treatments or generally when you feel the need.

As you use the Muin Essence, it will act as a catalyst between your energetic fields and those around you. This means that when somebody has your best interests at heart, they will receive abundance, love and joy. As you meet and mingle with those who mean you no harm or will do right by you, Muin offers healing, balance and harmony.

However, when you encounter those who in some way want to hurt, take from, or otherwise harm you, Muin becomes defensive and will offer a nasty sting. Some people report this to be like a bee-sting or very painful prickle at various locations in their body. Thus Muin is the ultimate in Celtic Reiki defences!

The important thing to remember with Muin is that you never use it to hurt or harm or to create joy or balance – you just use it. The essence will react with those you are connected to and it is the synthesis of Muin and their intent that creates the effect.

You will also find that the effects of Muin are only apparent whilst in your company, so if you use Muin and then encounter somebody who means you harm, they will only have the negative reactions to the essence whilst they are in your immediate space – as soon as they move to a distance where they cannot harm you, the effects will dissipate only to return if they come closer again.

Other aspects of Muin are loyalty, trust, friendship, reconciliation, abundance, prosperity, joy, happiness and the turning of the tides.

Physical: Diabetes and issues surrounding sugar. Also for hernia and health challenges regarding boundaries.

Emotional/Mental: Loyalty amongst friends, colleagues and loved-ones. Happiness and joy, especially when seeking a blissful attitude to one's daily approach to life.

Spiritual: Assertion in spiritual matters. Guardianship and gatekeepers.

The Oracle of Muin

"Darling!" she says. "Come rest a while!" for the Bramble curls her stems around you and before you know it you are bound by her prickly wiles. Loving and protective, the Muin essence is here to offer kindness and protection—she will guide you through rough patches and offer support in times of need – she offers sustenance in the form of sweet, juicy berries and a safe haven in her thorny branches.

There is also a darker side to the Blackberry, for as she creates her place of safety and shelter, food and support, she builds an enchantment wrapped in thorns. Is all in your current situation as it seems? Have you chosen to become wrapped up in an illusion for the sake of ease or comfort? Maybe you seek shelter, when you could be creating resolution—are you hiding when a proactive response is required? The Muin essence offers kindness and security for now, but do not get too comfortable, or you might experience entanglement in those thorns!

If you feel the need to defend, the Bramble will offer you a fortress, if you feel the need for recuperation, she will give rest and a harbour from the elements, if you need love, she will offer words of comfort and support.

What Muin also offers is a clear and definite reminder that whilst it is good to rest, to ask for help, and to take time for oneself, do not lose sight of your own abilities to be strong, create change, tackle challenges, and love oneself unconditionally. "Darling!" comes the cry. "Would you be an absolute dear and place your hands on my thorns!"—"Well, actually," you reply. "No, I'd rather not!"

GORT
IVY - G - [GORT]

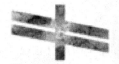

THERE ONCE WAS A TREE THAT HAD THE REPUTATION FOR BEING A LITTLE CHALLENGED IN THE INTELLIGENCE DEPARTMENT. THIS WAS A GREAT AMUSEMENT TO THE OTHER TREES IN THE WOODLAND, WHO WOULD ASK HIM TO DO SIMPLE SUMS AND THEN LAUGH RAUCOUSLY WHEN HE GOT THE ANSWERS WRONG. DURING ONE OF THESE BOUTS OF ROWDY GUFFAWING, AN ENCHANTED SPRITE WHO WAS TRYING TO TAME A WILD ZEPHYR, FELL UPON THEM.

"WHAT'S GOING ON?" SHE ASKED.

"WE ASKED THIS STUPID TREE WHAT TWO PLUS THREE IS AND HE ANSWERED, 'A HEDGEHOG'!" THE TREE REPLIED.

"WELL, TEASING A LITTLE TREE LIKE THAT IS NOT VERY NICE!" THE SPRITE CHIDED, WITH HER HANDS ON HER HIPS. "I FEEL THAT YOU ALL NEED TO BE GIVEN A CHALLENGE OF YOUR OWN TO DEAL WITH!"

AND WITH THAT, THERE WAS A FLASH OF SPARKLY LIGHT AND THE MATHEMATICALLY CHALLENGED TREE STARTED TO GROWN MANY, MANY BRANCHES. THESE THIN, CURLY TENDRILS BEGAN TO WEAVE THEIR WAY UP THE TRUNKS OF THE TREES AND UP, INTO THEIR BRANCHES.

"NOW, WHENEVER YOU NEED TO ANSWER A QUESTION OF NUMBERS," THE SPRITE EXPLAINED TO THE NEWLY-TRANSFORMED TREE. "YOU CAN USE YOUR BRANCHES TO KEEP COUNT!"

SINCE THAT DAY, GORT HAS BECOME VERY ADEPT AT ANSWERING QUESTIONS, NOT ONLY OF NUMBERS, BUT OF ANY SUBJECT AND LEVEL OF COMPLEXITY. HOWEVER, WHENEVER A TREE ASKS FOR ADVICE, THEY MUST REPAY GORT'S TIME, BY ALLOWING HIM TO GROW ON THEM IN RETURN.

Gort is the perspective of the Ivy and is connected to the cerebral and psychological. The ivy creates a labyrinth – a tangle of paths and journeys. Some lead you forward, some lead you to nowhere, some lead you round and round. The Gort Essence will help you to find your way through the labyrinth, helping you to stick to the right path.

Gort can help to manifest clarity, improve memory and help you connect to higher wisdom.

He can calm the mind in times of anxiety and allow stillness in meditation. You can use Gort if you wish to manifest anonymously for the higher good, i.e., you know you need something, but you are not quite sure what.

Gort was also the second Homœopathic remedy created in the Celtic Tree range, created from a large plant located in Central London.

Physical: Acts mainly on the heart for cardiac disorders. A good hangover cure!

Emotional/Mental: Confusion or those who feel lost. Mental haze or an overactive mind – creates stillness and focus. The Gort Essence will help you to find your way through the labyrinth, helping you to stick to the right path. Gort can help to manifest clarity, improve memory and help you connect to higher wisdom.

Spiritual: The main aspect of this frequency is that of spiritual enlightenment, of finding and sticking to one's path. It can free the spirit and unify energy to create a single purpose or it can branch out and raise the spirit to give a new perspective of the wider picture.

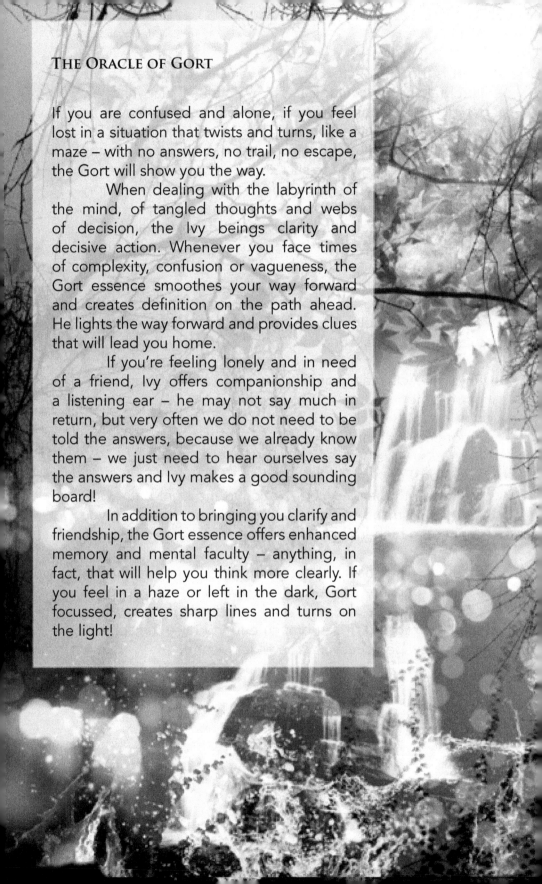

THE ORACLE OF GORT

If you are confused and alone, if you feel lost in a situation that twists and turns, like a maze – with no answers, no trail, no escape, the Gort will show you the way.

When dealing with the labyrinth of the mind, of tangled thoughts and webs of decision, the Ivy beings clarity and decisive action. Whenever you face times of complexity, confusion or vagueness, the Gort essence smoothes your way forward and creates definition on the path ahead. He lights the way forward and provides clues that will lead you home.

If you're feeling lonely and in need of a friend, Ivy offers companionship and a listening ear – he may not say much in return, but very often we do not need to be told the answers, because we already know them – we just need to hear ourselves say the answers and Ivy makes a good sounding board!

In addition to bringing you clarify and friendship, the Gort essence offers enhanced memory and mental faculty – anything, in fact, that will help you think more clearly. If you feel in a haze or left in the dark, Gort focussed, creates sharp lines and turns on the light!

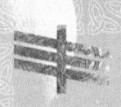

NGETAL
BROOM|NETTLE
NG - [NET-TARL]

THERE ONCE WAS A TREE WITH A RATHER PECULIAR HABIT. THIS HABIT WAS SO UNUSUAL IN THE REALM OF TREES THAT MANY WOULD BLUSH AT THE MERE MENTION OF IT. THE TREE'S NEIGHBOURS WOULD HIDE IN SHAME FOR MERELY BEING IN THE PROXIMITY OF SUCH STRANGE AND UNSOCIAL BEHAVIOUR. PASSING TRAVELLERS WOULD OFTEN STOP AND LOOK SIDE-LONG AT THE TREE; THEY WOULD TURN THEIR HEADS TO A CERTAIN POINT, GO GOOGLE-EYED AND THEN RUN OFF IN SHOCK.

IT WAS NOT LONG BEFORE THE TREES BEGAN TO HANG THEIR HEADS IN DESPAIR, NOT QUITE KNOWING WHAT TO DO. EVENTUALLY THEY DECIDED TO CALL UPON THE HORNED ONE TO RESOLVE THE SITUATION. HE ANSWERED THEIR CALL AND CAME TO SEE WHAT ALL THE FUSS WAS ABOUT. WHEN HE ARRIVED, HE STOOD IN FRONT OF THE TREE AND GAZED FOR A WHILE, NOT SURE WHAT HE WAS SEEING. HE TURNED HIS HEAD SLOWLY TO THE LEFT IN AN ATTEMPT TO CLARIFY THE GOINGS-ON.

THE TREES WATCHED AS CERNUNNOS SEEMED MORE AND MORE PERPLEXED.

"AND JUST ABOUT NOW..." THEY CRIED AS HIS HEAD REACHED JUST THE RIGHT PLACE. THE HORNED ONE'S EYES NEARLY POPPED OUT OF HIS HEAD AND HE GASPED IN HORROR.

"THIS WILL NEVER DO!" HE WHISPERED AND IT WAS DONE.

THE OTHER TREES WATCHED AS THE TREE CONTINUED WITH HIS UNSAVOURY HABIT, BUT ALL OF A SUDDEN SOMETHING INCREDIBLE HAPPENED: THE TREE SPLIT IN TWO. HE STOPPED FOR A MOMENT, GATHERED HIS THOUGHTS AND THEN CONTINUED. NOW HE SPLIT INTO FOUR, THEN EIGHT, THEN SIXTEEN. EACH TIME HE STARTED TO ACT HABITUALLY, HIS TRUNK WOULD SPLIT RIGHT DOWN THE MIDDLE.

IT WAS NOT LONG BEFORE THERE WAS NO TRUNK, JUST MANY LONG BRANCHES THAT JUTTED FROM THE GROUND. IT WAS THEN THAT THE TREE STOPPED COMPLETELY AND SIMPLY BECAME VERY QUIET. WHEN HE REMAINED QUIET FOR LONG ENOUGH, FLOWERS WOULD GROW ON HIS BRANCHES, BUT IF EVER HE DARED TO RETURN TO HIS OLD WAYS, ALL HIS BRANCHES WOULD SPLIT IN TWO ONCE MORE. AND THAT WAS HOW NGETAL ENDED UP WITH ALL BRANCH AND NO TRUNK!

Ngetal is an excellent essence when dealing with excess and habitual behaviour, working on the levels of self-regulation and a deeper understanding of what is beneficial to health and what causes harm.

Often associated with royalty, this plant essence has a very 'regal' feel and is excellent for raising a person's perception to a more expansive level, rather like Ailim, but here the emphasis is on a higher perspective of the self and one's own behaviour rather than a situation based outlook.

A general cleansing and healing 'tonic', Ngetal works on the bladder, kidneys and lymphatic system, causing detoxification through its diuretic qualities. It purges the body of substances that are harmful to health, including toxic chemicals/vibrations that the focus has been exposed to during addictive behaviour; alcohol, smoking, drugs, etc.

In the Celtic calendar, Ngetal symbolises the end of summer and the onset of the winter months, thus ushering in a time of taking stock and reconciliation. This is also seen in the Ngetal Essence, as it helps a person reconcile recent events, learn from situations and past mistakes thus enabling them to move beyond what has happened.

The cycle of sleep in order to start anew with revitalised energy reserves and a fresh, positive attitude, is also seen in Ngetal as it is the essence equivalent of hibernation, offering the subject a chance to awaken from their treatment with newfound vigour and be completely energised. It can also create deep, restful slumber when a person is stressed or working too hard.

Using Ngetal could produce a narcoleptic effect on the treatment couch and this should be noted when using it. The focus of the treatment (or Practitioner) may also find the essence nurtures them to a place where they can put down things they cling to and drop the baggage they are carrying.

The narcotic effects of Ngetal can also be used in sleep disorders – those who cannot sleep or those who are lethargic and sleep too much. The essence will help find balance and a natural, healthy routine of peaceful sleep and energised daily activity. Ngetal will help those who work shifts and have irregular sleep patterns and thus a confused 'body-clock'.

Remember, however, that the essence works towards the benefit of your health and not your working objectives, so if you are dangerously over-tired, Ngetal could send you to sleep so that you get a much-needed recharge, rather than helping you to stay awake further!

The Celtic Reiki Ngetal Essence was harvested from two individuals who were rescued from a discount garden centre that was badly mistreating and neglecting their plants.

The two Broom plants were near to death and crying out to passers-by in a last attempt to be saved. Once rescued, both Broom plants made a remarkable recovery and are now fully back to health, wildly energetic and have even seeded!

Physical: The bladder, urinary tract, kidneys, and lymphatic system. Excellent detoxifier and cleansing essence. Creates a clearing effect on the body and fluids of the body, such as blood, water, etc. Over-indulgence in food, alcohol, etc. Sleep disorders, ME and lethargy are also treated with Ngetal

Emotional/Mental: Taking stock of a project or period in one's life as it approaches fruition. Perhaps when one is facing a point where tough decisions need to be made about whether a project (or path) is worth continuing with. Reconciliation and consolidation.

Spiritual: Energy, vibrancy, power.

THE ORACLE OF NGETAL

The delicate, dark green stems of the broom gently caress your cheek and you open your eyes to her beautiful, yellow blooms. She speaks and her voice is soft and kind. She has come to fill your life with her essence and as she wraps her influence into the paths, dynamics and actions you take, you will begin to see things from another perspective.

For Ngetal offers insight into the self-sabotaging steps you are taking, without even knowing it. She offers insight into your habitual patterns that are so ingrained into your view of the world that you barely notice them any more – she enables you to cleanse, to reconcile and to take stock of what has come before, perchance you may recognise your habits and change them.

The Broom's tranquil essence, is not strong or vibrant, like her cousin the Gorse, yet it is in this gentleness that her power lies. For as she blows gentle kisses to you, there will come a clarity that you have never before seen – deceit will become apparent, sabotage clear, and you will understand your life without the blinkers of character that hide you from the truth of any situation.

And once you've witnessed the patterns and behaviours you have, in the past, employed to negate your dreams and success, Ngetal will be by your side as you repattern and alter your actions. She will guide you to a path where every choice and step leads you to your dreams. And once you have spent a day achieving every joy your heart desires, fulfilling wishes and learning how to be the best you can be, she will help you sleep – for Broom is the essence of a good night's sleep and very sweet dreams – so as you drift off in a tranquil slumber, you will begin to dream once again, enchanted dreams that lead you onwards to new adventures, new dreams and desires for the new day to come.

STRAIF
BLACKTHORN - ST - [STRIFE]

A TREE LOOKED OUT INTO THE WORLD AND SAW A PLACE OF CRUELTY AND PAIN. THIS CAUSED THE TREE SO MUCH DISTRESS THAT HIS VERY BEING STARTED TO DEADEN. IN AN ATTEMPT TO BLOCK OUT THE TERRIBLE THINGS HE HAD WITNESSED, HE GREW GIANT THORNS TO WARD OFF OTHERS, BUT STILL THE MOST SHOCKING EVENTS OF THE WORLD CAME TO HIM.

THE TREE THEN TRIED TO CURL UP INTO THE SMALLEST PLACE HE COULD, BECOMING DENSE AND CROOKED. YET, STILL HE COULD HEAR WORDS OF HATE AND CRIES OF WAR. HE CALLED TO GRANDMOTHER SUN TO HELP HIM, BUT STILL THE EMOTIONS OF ANGER AND GRIEF WERE ALL AROUND HIM, MAKING HIS SKIN THE DARKEST BLACK AND HIS BERRIES, BITTER.

VERY SOON, THE EFFECTS WERE SO OBVIOUS THAT HE BECAME KNOWN AS 'STRIFE' AND ALL WOULD GIVE HIM A WIDE BERTH.

ONE STORMY NIGHT, A LITTLE ORPHAN CAME AND SHELTERED UNDER THE THORNY BRANCHES OF STRAIF. AT FIRST THE TREE TRIED TO SEND THE ORPHAN AWAY, BUT SHE WAS SO FRIGHTENED THAT THE GRUMPY-OLD TREE LET HER STAY. IN THE MORNING, WHEN THE STORM HAD PASSED AND THE LITTLE GIRL WAS READY TO GO ON HER WAY, SHE THANKED HIM FOR GIVING HER SHELTER. AS SHE WISHED HIM WELL, HIS BRANCHES BURST FORTH WITH THE MOST BEAUTIFUL WHITE BLOSSOM AND HE FELT JOY.

FROM THEN ON, STRAIF HELPS THOSE WHO NEED SHELTER AND ADVICE, FOR NOTHING MAKES THE PAIN OF THE WORLD DISAPPEAR LIKE A SMALL ACT OF KINDNESS...

As the name suggests, the essence of Straif releases us from the trouble and strife that we encounter in our everyday lives. In many ways, Straif acts as a tonic, but it works on deeper levels than just those needed to soothe and calm – the Blackthorn perspective counteracts and releases all areas of darkness and pain in our lives.

Straif could be seen as a rescue remedy, as it helps those in real need; the people who can see no way out of the despair they find themselves in. It offers emergency light to what appears to be unending darkness.

Blackthorn, despite its reputation, is such a beautiful tree; the black bark and stunning blossom make it one of the most joyous celebrations of the spring, arriving before most other trees come into flower.

When used in a treatment, this element of Straif can be useful for it can be placed into a treatment just before Huathe, in order to create an even deeper result when clearing the suppressed and hidden trauma that we spend most of our lives trying to run away from and not acknowledging as part of us.

Physical: Comforts the suicidal and the lost. People who self-harm or have attempted to take their life.

Emotional/Mental: Straif supports us in our conflicts and troubles – not just the challenges we face from time to time, but the really horrific strife that we may come across only once or twice. The Straif essence is the most wonderful essence when working with the obstacles that threaten to derail us. From hatred, vengeance, slander, libel, hate campaigns and being judged unfairly, Straif will give the strength to go on.

Spiritual: Straif could be seen as a rescue remedy, as it helps those in real need; the people who can see no way out of the despair they find themselves in.

THE ORACLE OF STRAIF

When Straif arrives in any reading, it is usually because you have experienced or are experiencing times of utter pain and anguish. These times often feel utterly hopeless, without hope of letting up or release from the torment you have known.

Yet is not the strife of his name this essence comes to offer you—it is transcendence of pain and trauma that the Blackthorn presents to you. His wondrous gift will completely wash away your pain to such an extent, it will be as if that old life never existed. You will view the world like a child again.

The essence of Straif is like a summer's day of warm air and blue skies, lush green plants and an abundance of wildlife.

Here is the joy of creation and being born anew—however this is a rebirth, in which everything you were, everything you have achieved and learnt is still within you—but like a caterpillar, the Blackthorn essence will guide you to your own blissful rest in a place of stasis—your own chrysalis. From which you will eventually burst into life, a new life, where anything can be yours and will be.

During this stasis, take time to focus on what is to come. The desires you have, the achievements you want to strive for, and the details of goals you have yet to achieve.

Plan for a big adventure; a wonder-filled voyage of self-discovery and complete attainment. Create as a child would create—with excitement, anticipation and complete commitment to this moment. "Soon will come the time for you to be anew, so use this time well," the Blackthorn says.

RUIS
ELDER - R - [RWEESH]

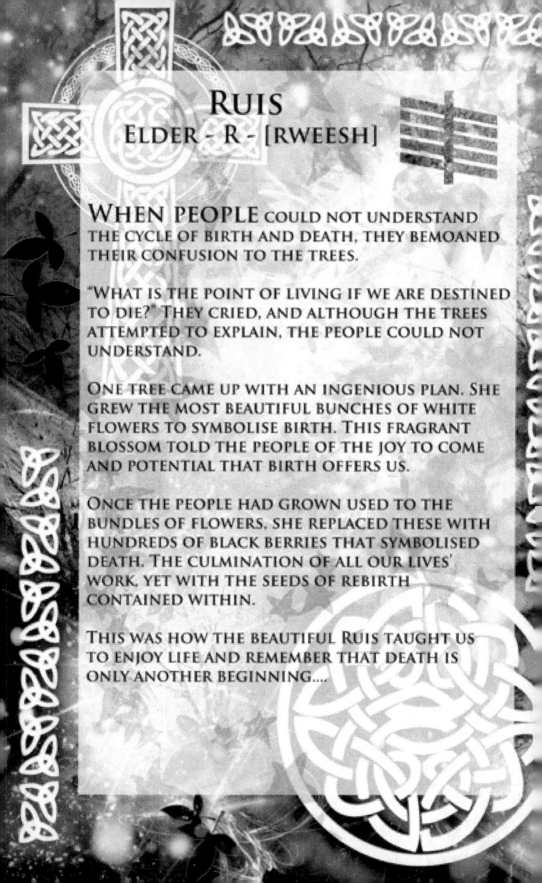

WHEN PEOPLE COULD NOT UNDERSTAND THE CYCLE OF BIRTH AND DEATH, THEY BEMOANED THEIR CONFUSION TO THE TREES.

"WHAT IS THE POINT OF LIVING IF WE ARE DESTINED TO DIE?" THEY CRIED, AND ALTHOUGH THE TREES ATTEMPTED TO EXPLAIN, THE PEOPLE COULD NOT UNDERSTAND.

ONE TREE CAME UP WITH AN INGENIOUS PLAN. SHE GREW THE MOST BEAUTIFUL BUNCHES OF WHITE FLOWERS TO SYMBOLISE BIRTH. THIS FRAGRANT BLOSSOM TOLD THE PEOPLE OF THE JOY TO COME AND POTENTIAL THAT BIRTH OFFERS US.

ONCE THE PEOPLE HAD GROWN USED TO THE BUNDLES OF FLOWERS, SHE REPLACED THESE WITH HUNDREDS OF BLACK BERRIES THAT SYMBOLISED DEATH. THE CULMINATION OF ALL OUR LIVES' WORK, YET WITH THE SEEDS OF REBIRTH CONTAINED WITHIN.

THIS WAS HOW THE BEAUTIFUL RUIS TAUGHT US TO ENJOY LIFE AND REMEMBER THAT DEATH IS ONLY ANOTHER BEGINNING....

Ruis is the essence of the Elder Tree and is the perspective of birth and death, the beginning and the end. This essence allows us knowledge of the cycle of life and can be used at any time of loss and transition, including the journey beyond life.

In treatments, Ruis can also be used at the beginning of any session that involves dealing with deeply embedded issues that might trigger a fear reaction or deep emotional/physical pain. When treated it will help the person to cope with these symptoms of the clearing.

In manifestation rituals, Ruis is excellent for issues surrounding the law and legal disputes. It will always work with respect for natural law, so cannot be used to sway the outcome. However, if you feel that you or your client is likely to lose the argument, it can help an amicable result to be reached, thus releasing severe loss.

The Ruis Essence is excellent for those who are 'too' grounded. For example, those who focus on the physical and on material possessions or things. Ruis will lift them up to 'free' their mind and spirit and then gently ground them again, so they land in a much healthier place!

Physical: Works particularly well on sore throats or infections of the throat. The stomach is another area that would benefit from Ruis. The essence can also help with arthritis, rheumatism and sciatica.

Emotional/Mental: Will help the bereaved or those who have lost and need to grow before they can move on. Fear generally and especially fear of change.

Spiritual: Offers acceptance of one's life path, even if the person resists strongly at first – it can even create a zest for the future on a spirit's journey.

THE ORACLE OF RUIS

The soft, delicate essence of Ruis wafts on the breeze and into your life like an aroma, caught for a moment and then gone. At times when he is with you, you breathe deeply in an attempt to savour every sensory explosion of his being, pulling his scent deep within you and when he is gone, his memory defies words, transcends definition. For Ruis is a gift—a momentary, transitory spark of inspiration, of enlightenment, of freedom from the things that hold you back.

When you are aware of the Elder's presence it is often because you are in some troublesome situation, maybe a legal dispute or some form of disagreement with another person, maybe you feel paralysed with fear as to your next move, maybe you find yourself treated unfairly or accused of what you have not done, or maybe you have suffered unbearable loss.

Whatever the whys and wherefores of your situation, the Elder gently reminds you that you may be too grounded into the world of definition and this could be the root of your pain.

He says that you are of the Earth and all the joys of the Earth, but this 'world' you believe to be real, is merely a definition, thought up by other people. It is no more real than any thought, or any definition. To be grounded in the Earth offers strength, courage and an essential feeling of connection and bliss. To be overly grounded in the world of human definition is often to lose your vital connection to Earth and to believe that what is the will of others is important.

Yet, remember—when others define the world, they speak only of themselves—if they hate, it is because they find themselves in hate; if they accuse, the accusation is for themselves; if they tell you it will be horrible, it is because they fear the consequences themselves. None of these are your thoughts—so let them go, connect to the Earth and rediscover your own will, your own perspective of the Earth and let Ruis guide you through your difficulties.

UILLEAND
HONEYSUCKLE - PE - [OO-LIND]

A TREE THAT IS BORN INTO SHADOW HAS LITTLE CHANCE OF A FULL LIFE, YET STILL THEY FOCUS, EACH DAY, ON ACHIEVING AS MUCH AS THEY CAN WITH WHAT THEY HAVE. A LIFETIME IN THE DARKNESS, WITH LITTLE LIGHT AND GROUND THAT HAS BEEN SUCKED CLEAN OF MANY NUTRIENTS. YET THE PROSPECT OF THIS, DID NOT STOP ONE DETERMINED INDIVIDUAL.

SHE KEPT HER BRANCHES THIN, WRAPPING THEM AROUND THE TRUNKS OF THOSE WHO CAME BEFORE HER. SHE USED THEIR STRENGTH TO SUPPORT HER AND MAINTAINED HER SIGHTS ON CLIMBING AS HIGH AS SHE COULD. EACH DAY SHE FOUGHT, NOT ONLY TO SURVIVE, BUT TO LIBERATE HERSELF FROM THE BLACKNESS OF THE FOREST FLOOR.

EVENTUALLY, SHE CLIMBED SO HIGH THAT SHE ENTWINED HERSELF AROUND THE BRANCHES OF HER ELDERS AND PUSHED HER LEAVES INTO THE BRILLIANT SUNLIGHT, ABOVE THE CANOPY. HERE SHE WAS ABLE TO BASK IN THE LIGHT AND GROW BEAUTIFUL, SCENTED FLOWERS THAT FILLED THE AIR WITH THEIR AROMA.

FROM THAT DAY ONWARDS, THE PERFUME OF UILLEAND REMINDS US THAT IF WE ARE DETERMINED, WE CAN CLIMB TO ANY HEIGHT AND DO ANYTHING, EVEN IF IT SEEMS IMPOSSIBLE.

One thing that is striking about the Honeysuckle is its ability to survive through trauma, yet not through being strong or battling its way forward.

Honeysuckle overcomes adversity through beauty, love and sweetness—the light of the Uilleand Essence reflects this and enables us to put down the 'fight' and the 'struggle', helping us to go forward and overcome our difficulties by shining with a light so bright that we can wash away darkness and shadow, working from within as opposed to fixing blame externally.

Truth comes from within us, as does fear – there is nothing outside of us that is more frightening than that which lurks within. In fact we can only be scared of things that exist within us, for, if we do not have the potential to be that thing that scares us, we cannot connect to it!

If you are afraid of the dark, it is because there is darkness within you. If you are afraid of being alone, it is because you have that loneliness within yourself and if you are frightened of being hurt, it is because you have the ability to hurt others. Uilleand enables us to see past the externalisation of our fears. She helps us to go inside and shine light upon our darkest, inaccessible parts.

This does not mean the process is a struggle or even painful, for Uilleand will help us overcome these difficulties through positive steps and healthy assertion of who we truly are. Natural command, ease of being and the conviction of walking forward with a smile are all signs of this essence and will enable someone to be much stronger than they thought they could be.

Physical: Lower abdominal issues, thyroid and throat dis-ease.

Emotional/Mental: Lethargy, depression and generally feeling 'low' are all eased by Honeysuckle. Fizzy and vibrant, she creates laughter, social bonds and motivation to tackle what must be done.

Spiritual: Spiritual understanding and creativity. Helps us to express spiritual concepts through creation and art, as well as assisting us in understanding a spiritual ethos that is unclear, paradoxical or dogmatic.

OIR
SPINDLE - TH - [U-EH]

"PUMPKINS ARE THE FINEST THINGS!"
SAID THE TREE THAT LIVED NEXT TO A HUGE PUMPKIN PATCH.

EACH YEAR HE WOULD WATCH AS THE PEOPLE FROM A NEARBY VILLAGE WOULD COME UP TO THE PATCH AND CELEBRATE THE HARVEST OF THE PLUMPEST, TASTIEST PUMPKINS YOU EVER DID SEE. THEN, IN THE SPRING, THEY WOULD RETURN AND PLANT THE SEEDS FROM THE PREVIOUS YEAR. THE PEOPLE SEEMED SO HAPPY AND JOYOUS, AS DID THE PUMPKIN PATCH, WHO WAS ALWAYS SO PLEASED TO SEE THE BELOVED VILLAGERS.

THE TREE DECIDED TO GROW PUMPKINS ALSO, IN THE HOPE THAT THE PEOPLE OF THE VILLAGE WOULD VISIT HIM AND PLANT HIS SEEDS ALSO. HE TRIED AND TRIED AND WHEN AUTUMN CAME, LITTLE PINK PUMPKINS BURST FROM HIS BRANCHES. THESE LOVELY LITTLE BERRIES WERE VERY PRETTY, BUT NOT BIG ENOUGH OR TASTY ENOUGH FOR THE VILLAGERS. SO THE TREE SPENT ANOTHER YEAR WATCHING ALONE, AS THE PUMPKIN BECAME THE CENTRE OF THE PEOPLE'S AFFECTION.

THE NEXT YEAR, THE TREE HAD AN IDEA - IN EACH PINK PUMPKIN-SHAPED SEED, HE WOULD PLACE A GIFT WITHIN FOR THOSE WHO PLANTED THE SEEDS. THIS WAS INCITEMENT ENOUGH FOR THE VILLAGERS, WHO STARTED TO COME AND PICK HIS BERRIES. THEY WOULD MAKE A WISH AND THEN PLANT THE SEEDS, SO THAT AS THE NEW TREES GREW, THEIR WISHES WOULD COME TRUE.

SOON, THE TREE CAME TO BE KNOWN AS OIR, THE MASTER OF DREAMS COME TRUE AND FULFILLED WISHES...

Oir is the Spindle, of sweetness and delight, and is used in Celtic Reiki to manifest an ideal situation. This could be more prosperity, a better job or a strengthening of relationships. Oir will help to create a conducive outcome in a physical sense and therefore is best used where money, property, work or people are concerned.

Another aspect of the Spindle is that of reward. It is for those who work hard, but receive no gratitude or thanks and also for those who expect reward for everything they do.

Spindle helps us carry out the tasks we must do, not for want or promise of reward, but because we should enjoy them and for the lessons we learn in the undertaking. It helps us to appreciate the journey we take rather than concentrating on the destination at the end of it.

Physical: Muscular pain and spasms. Issues with the left-hand-side of the body, particularly the shoulder, arm and hand. Cold sores and sores of the eyes, nose and mouth. Acne on forehead and back.

Emotional/Mental: Relationships, especially when attempting a reconciliation or reunion. Helps integrate knowledge and wisdom.

Spiritual: The learning of spiritual lessons.

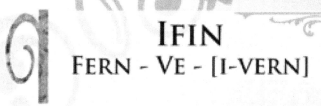

IFIN
FERN - VE - [I-VERN]

A TREE ONCE DECIDED

THAT THE OTHER TREES OF THE WOODLAND
REALM SPENT FAR TOO MUCH TIME REACHING FOR
THE SKY, WHEN SOME PLANTS WERE ABLE TO LIVE
JUST AS HAPPILY IN THE SHADY, MOIST, NOOKS AND
CRANNIES OF THE UNDERGROWTH. IT SEEMED
STRANGE TO HIM THAT SO MANY WOULD SPEND
SUCH A LARGE PROPORTION OF THEIR LIVES
WORKING SO HARD TO GET TALLER THAN EACH
OTHER.

SO THE TREE WRAPPED HIMSELF UP INTO A SMALL
BALL OF GREEN AND SPENT THE LONG WINTER
MONTHS CREATING INNER-CHANGE -
TRANSFORMING HIMSELF INTO A LITTLE TREE THAT
COULD SURVIVE IN THE PLACES WHERE LARGER
TREES WOULD SIMPLY DIE.

WHEN THE SPRING CAME, HE UNWRAPPED HIS
NEW BRANCHES - DELICATE FEATHERS OF GREEN
SPLAYED OUT FROM THE ROOTS OF TREES. FOR
A GLORIOUS SUMMER HE WAS ADMIRED BY THE
OTHER PLANTS AND CREATURES OF THE
WOODLAND, BUT WHEN THE WINTER APPROACHED,
HE KNEW IT WAS TIME TO CURL BACK UP INTO A
BALL AND WAIT FOR THE SUNSHINE TO RETURN.

NOW HIS CHILDREN GROW EACH YEAR ON
HEDGEROWS AND IN SHELTERED GLADES, THEY
DECORATE THE FOREST FLOOR AND ROCKY
STREAMS. THEY ARE KNOWN AS IFIN; THOSE WHO
FIND THE MIDDLE GROUND!

Added to the Celtic Reiki System in 2006, Ifin is a welcome addition to the essence canon, as Ferns are one of the most prolific and omnipresent plants to be seen in the Celtic lands today. Decorating the hedgerows, ferns are happiest in the shade of the other trees, which protect from the harsh light of the summer sun. This is reflected in the use of Ifin Essence.

Ifin can be used wherever the brightness of a treatment creates trauma or pain – this may seem like a misnomer, yet some people are affected painfully during or after the treatment. For those who find the healing process creates clearings or detoxifications that are too much to bear, Ifin will soften the effects and ease the healing process.

Ifin will also soften the 'edges' wherever you encounter a situation that is black and white, enabling the perception of the shades of grey that lie in between.

Physical: Burns and photosensitivity.

Emotional/Mental: Emotional and psychological pain and anguish. Helps those who cannot cope.

Spiritual: Helps alleviate the "I'm right, you're wrong" attitude, especially in spiritual circles, psychic groups, and other expanded arenas.

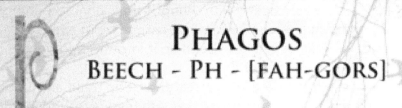

PHAGOS
BEECH - PH - [FAH-GORS]

FOR MANY MILLENNIA...

TREES AND MEN HAVE LIVED TOGETHER AND HAD MANY INTERACTIONS. THEY HAVE SUPPORTED EACH OTHER AND SHOWN KINDNESS WHEN THE OTHER NEEDED IT. HOWEVER, WHEN THE TREES DECIDED NEVER TO WRITE THINGS DOWN, FOR FEAR OF THE HUMANS TAKING ADVANTAGE OF THEIR WORDS, IT FELL UPON ONE TREE TO KEEP ALL THE IMPORTANT WISDOM OF TREES. EVERYTHING THE TREES HAD WRITTEN, BEFORE THE BETRAYAL OF PEOPLE, WAS PLACED INSIDE THIS TREE AND PASSED ON THROUGH THE SAP-LINE TO HER CHILDREN AND GRANDCHILDREN.

WHEN THE EARTH APPROACHED A TIME OF GREAT CHANCE AND PEOPLE BEGAN TO LEARN THE ERROR OF THEIR BEHAVIOUR (BOTH CURRENT AND ANCESTRAL), THE CHILDREN OF PHAGOS STARTED TO READ FROM THEIR INTERNAL SCRIPTS, SO ALL THE TREES OF THE WOODLAND REALM COULD, ONCE AGAIN, LEARN HOW TO LOVE AND INTERACT WITH HUMANS.

SO WHEN THE PEOPLE WERE READY TO LEARN ANCIENT WISDOM, FROM A NEW PERSPECTIVE, THE TREES HAD A RECORD OF WHERE TO BEGIN...

Working so extensively with Phagos has enabled the creation of not just one Beech Tree essence, but two. The essence of Phagos has now been split into the traditional Beech tree, and Copper Beech.

Beech is one of the most energetic trees and its vibrancy can be felt very strongly whether you are working with the youngest of saplings or the greatest of trees. The tree of wisdom and written knowledge is an interesting paradox for a race of people who did not write down their secrets, using the written word for communication and artistic purposes rather than wisdom.

To have a tree that symbolises a concept, non-existent in its culture, offers us a new twist to the traditional Phagos Essence: to understand what cannot be and yet is. The Old Lore; a fluid verbal tradition that is older than Wiccan and Druidic faiths, is never written down.

Hence it is very rare and is now scarcely used, but it teaches us that when information is written down, it is fixed at that point—unchanging. It can therefore become dogma and so no longer has a place in Old Lore, which constantly changes and evolves and is added to.

To remain fluid and based upon experience, instead of rules and 'facts', the tradition of Old Lore has to be passed down verbally from Master to Student – if ever you read any 'facts' about Old Lore, they are not Old Lore!

This is the essence of Phagos, for it symbolises written knowledge. Yet as soon as that knowledge is written, it stops being knowledge and becomes stagnant and limited. Phagos therefore provides us with the understanding of paradox and that which cannot be, for it contradicts itself.

Whenever faced with a situation or subject that is a mixture of coexisting opposites and contradictions, Phagos will help us to use what cannot be to make sense of what we encounter and shift it to our understanding.

We could say that the written knowledge of Phagos is writing that we have not encountered or cannot understand yet, but exists in a way that is outside our common knowledge—like a massive encyclopaedia of perspectives that we can use and interpret in our own way – this is written, but written in essence not in words. Perhaps Phagos can help us see other ways of solving the paradoxes of life?

Physical: Assimilation of food, excessive hunger, over-eating, eating disorders and obesity. Phagos can not only be used to help cut down on food consumption, but also to help nurture a healthy attitude towards nutrition, food and exercise.

Emotional/Mental: Cerebral activities, learning, reading and writing. The transmission of knowledge and expansion of the mind. Psychology and social dynamics.

Spiritual: The spirituality of the written word, memetics and higher beings.

LLOCHW
BLUEBELL - LL – [CLOCK-AU]

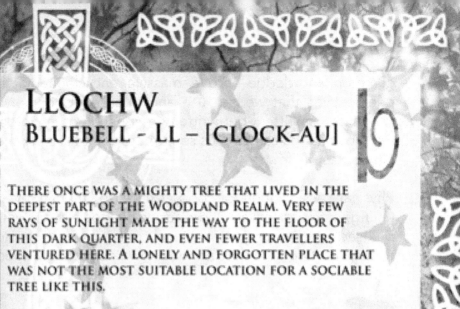

THERE ONCE WAS A MIGHTY TREE THAT LIVED IN THE DEEPEST PART OF THE WOODLAND REALM. VERY FEW RAYS OF SUNLIGHT MADE THE WAY TO THE FLOOR OF THIS DARK QUARTER, AND EVEN FEWER TRAVELLERS VENTURED HERE. A LONELY AND FORGOTTEN PLACE THAT WAS NOT THE MOST SUITABLE LOCATION FOR A SOCIABLE TREE LIKE THIS.

FOR A HUNDRED YEARS THE TREE GREW IN SIZE AND IN SADNESS. EVENTUALLY, AS THE PAIN GREW TO BE UNBEARABLE, THE TREE DECIDED THAT HE NO LONGER WANTED TO LIVE AND BEGAN TO CURL UP SMALLER AND SMALLER, HOPING TO DISAPPEAR INTO NOTHINGNESS.

FINALLY HE WAS CURLED UP SO SMALL THAT HE WAS NOTHING MORE THAN A SINGLE GREEN STEM AND FEW LEAVES. HE PULLED HIS LEAVES TOGETHER AND WRAPPED THEM INTO A SINGLE LITTLE FLOWER; A BEAUTIFUL, PURPLE-BLUE BELL THAT SHONE VIBRANTLY IN THE SINGLE RAY OF SUNLIGHT THAT MANAGED TO BREAK THROUGH THE CANOPY ABOVE.

THEN, SOMETHING REMARKABLE HAPPENED, FOR A LONE NOMAD, WHO JUST HAPPENED TO BE PASSING, SAW THIS PRETTY LITTLE FLOWER AND CAME AWAY FROM THE PATH TO GAZE UPON ITS BEAUTY.

IT WAS NOT LONG BEFORE OTHERS HEARD OF THIS BEAUTIFUL 'BLUE BELL' AND CAME TO SEE IT FOR THEMSELVES. THE TREE WAS SO HAPPY THAT HE WAS, AT LAST, LOVED THAT HE HAD A THOUSAND CHILDREN, WHO EACH HAD A THOUSAND MORE; FORMING CARPETS OF THE MOST SUMPTUOUSLY RICH PURPLE. THIS WAS THE GIFT OF LLOCHW: THE TREE THAT BECAME A FLOWER; A HIDDEN GIFT THAT WAS TUCKED WAY IN THE DEEPEST AND SOMETIMES DARKEST PARTS OF THE WOODLAND REALM.

The Bluebell is the perspective of hidden gifts and treasures that are unspoken of. These are not intentionally placed out of sight or mind, but simply forgotten. Therefore, the essence of Llochw is that of things lost in time, rather than space.

Nowhere are there treasures more hidden, than those we forget we have inside of us. Llochw helps us to remember those lost and fragmented parts of ourselves that we once took for granted and have since buried under mounds of trepidation and adult fears.

This essence is a call to action, a remembrance of who you were in a more innocent and happier time, before the (un-)reality of the world stopped you from taking chances and believing in who you could be—who you are.

The essence of Llochw also brings inner-beauty, hidden talents, and secret skills to the surface for us to reacquaint ourselves with. Hence, the perspective of the Bluebell can appear to transform who we are; actually, she just reminds us of who we have the potential to be, but had forgotten...

Physical: Hidden dis-ease and physical issues that are detectable through the symptoms they produce, but avoid diagnosis or direct detection.

Emotional/Mental: Ambivalence, or enigmatic emotional states—feelings of uncertainty, mixed emotions, confusion and conflicting thoughts. Victims, martyrs, or those who have no faith in themselves. Memory loss; be it dramatic or subtle.

Spiritual: Spiritual gifts and hidden abilities. Spiritual mysteries solved, new experiences brought to consciousness, old wonders reintegrated.

Rhywtawel
Rhododendron
Rh - (R-WHO-TAH-WELL)

As the world became filled with noise and radiation; as people ravaged the Earth's resources and chopped down forests to make cities; as the oceans became polluted and the creatures of the Earth suffered at human hands, one tree decided to make a difference. If he could create a place where all would be safe, no matter of creed or kind, then the Earth could become safe, once again.

So he burst into the most amazing display of colour, with flowers that bloomed so prolifically, so fragrantly that everyone who saw or smelled them, simply stopped and fell in love with the Earth, once again. Soon, the vibrant hues and perfumes of Rhywtawel formed a sanctuary that took away the hurt and embraced all who lived on the Earth. Soon, everything became harmonious.

But as Rhywtawel gave peace and joy to all, soaking up their fear and hatred, he began to die from all the pain and trauma he was saturated with. When he could take no more, he let all this emotion out through his roots and it poisoned the Earth, so that nothing could grow in the ground where his kind grow.

Thus, the gift of the Rhododendron became a conflicted one that gives us all a choice: to live a life, expecting others to make us happy, whilst pushing our pain into the Earth; to live in the shadow of trauma and hurt, carrying all our past challenges with us; or to find a balance that makes the experience the most heart-pounding, gut-wrenching ride it possibly can be...

The essence of Rhywtawel is a peaceful, tranquil perspective that lifts burdens and gently kisses away pain. It is a sanctuary unlike any other, for this is a place for the weary traveller to rest a while, but only for a while.

The Rhywtawel Essence reminds us that rest is essential, but so is the need to experience growth, action and adventure—to explore and create. Without these things, life is simply whiled away, rather than lived!

So, this perspective can help those who are at the end of their tether, or cannot face any more pain. It is also for those who are rested and need the motivation to start moving again. If you or your client have had the opportunity to take time out, such as a holiday or time of recuperation, and are finding it a challenge to gather speed, the essence of the Rhododendron will support the gathering of speed and energy.

Rhywtawel presents us with the choice to live fully or simply flop onto our knees and do nothing; he offers shelter to those who need it and a bitter taste to those who are reliant upon it. He invites us to deal with our trauma and release our pain in a responsible and autonomous away, thus taking blame out of any situation.

Physical: Lethargy, tiredness, exhaustion, ME, lack of strength or physical vitality. Coma or unconsciousness.

Emotional/Mental: No motivation or resistance to do what needs to be done—laziness or reliance on others. Those who blame others or refuse to take responsibility for themselves. People who seem to poison the things they come into contact with.

Spiritual: Empowerment and expansion, but also peace and serenity.

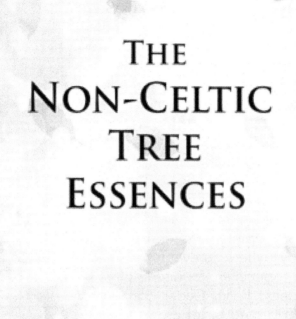

THE
NON-CELTIC
TREE
ESSENCES

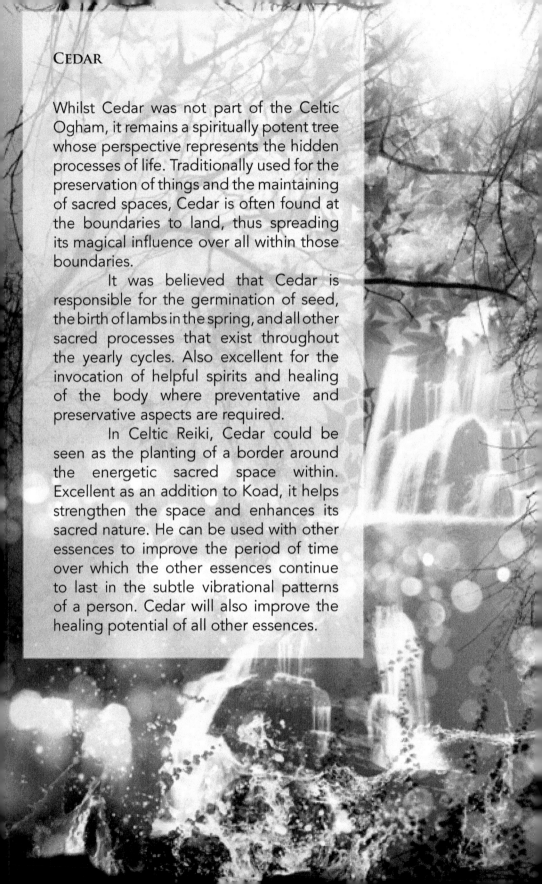

CEDAR

Whilst Cedar was not part of the Celtic Ogham, it remains a spiritually potent tree whose perspective represents the hidden processes of life. Traditionally used for the preservation of things and the maintaining of sacred spaces, Cedar is often found at the boundaries to land, thus spreading its magical influence over all within those boundaries.

It was believed that Cedar is responsible for the germination of seed, the birth of lambs in the spring, and all other sacred processes that exist throughout the yearly cycles. Also excellent for the invocation of helpful spirits and healing of the body where preventative and preservative aspects are required.

In Celtic Reiki, Cedar could be seen as the planting of a border around the energetic sacred space within. Excellent as an addition to Koad, it helps strengthen the space and enhances its sacred nature. He can be used with other essences to improve the period of time over which the other essences continue to last in the subtle vibrational patterns of a person. Cedar will also improve the healing potential of all other essences.

When used as a single essence, Cedar can be good at maintaining health in a preventative light, ensuring a greater resistance to disease and emotional trauma when used regularly. Cedar will also instil a sense of the 'body as a temple' within the subject, enabling them to view their physical form as a sacred receptacle in which their spirit is housed.

Cedar can also increase the life of things such as foodstuff, water, etc., preserving it and thus staving off decay for a greater length of time. With Cedar essence placed around the borders of your home and workspace, you create boundaries that, as people pass over them, they come to understand the sacred nature of your environment and become more respectful of it.

On physical levels, Cedar works well with the skin and conditions of the skin, such as psoriasis, cold sores (herpes), eczema, cuts and wounds, warts, pimples, acne and so on. It is excellent as a tonic for any disease that involves the deterioration or failure of physiological systems such as osteoporosis, liver cirrhosis, Alzheimer's Disease, renal failure, nervous breakdown and so on.

SYCAMORE

Sycamore is the essence of regeneration and endurance, the ability to last, whatever the situation and however long it goes on for. Excellent as a supportive and strengthening tonic when resolve is failing as it boosts and revitalises.

Sycamore provides answers when things have gone seriously wrong! Sycamore is not like Duir, who is strong and secure through sheer physical and energetic power—Sycamore gets her abilities elsewhere.

For she is one of the most susceptible to storms and bad weather, breaking in the wind and falling to Earth, yet she is able to repair herself very quickly and can grow back faster than the repeated storms can pull her down.

Therefore sycamore offers her support by enabling the subject to bounce back from trauma and this is excellent for all of us in times when we are knocked off our feet by something unexpected or unforeseen.

So if you are aware of an issue that needs strength and support, use Duir. However when the situation sneaks up on you and is upon you before you realise it, Sycamore is the essence to use—she will help you get back on to your feet very quickly and become more than you were before because of the trials you have faced.

ELM

Elm is a fascinating and much maligned essence that has now been reintroduced for healing use. Elm was actually one of the sacred Celtic Trees. This was sometimes quoted as Fearn, sometimes as Ailim, the latter being more likely due to the name (Ailim/Elm). The connotations of Elm are very dark indeed by modern standards, yet very useful if we are truthful with ourselves.

The appearance of Dutch Elm disease means this tragic species of tree rarely lives beyond the age of 30 years old, so it is destined to die young. Now scarce in Celtic areas of Britain and Europe, the Elm Essence has been harvested almost completely from cultivated species, as only one wild tree could be found.

The Elm was used a marker by the Celts for areas prone to disease, ill fortune or 'darkness': if the land were seen as 'bad', Elms would be planted to ward off others and act as a warning. This soon gave Elm the reputation of being about darkness and depression as well as inviting in bad-luck. This is perhaps why Elm's karma has been so tragic and painful to behold.

From the early origination of Celtic Reiki the perspective of a sick Elm was harvested and present in the essence repertoire (he was standing in close proximity to the Mid-Wales Oaks that originally comprised the Duir Essence).

This essence was not originally listed or used in Orientation, however, firstly because of the Elm being removed from 'popular Celtic belief', and also due to the implications of including a sick tree. After many trials and with several successful outcomes using essences from diseased or dying trees, this Elm is now included, along with the perspective of many other Elms.

Elm is indeed surrounded by bad luck and depression, yet as a physical being he acts as a magnet, drawing this ill fortune towards himself and away from others – he acts as a guide to the location and appearance of 'darkness' and malignancy.

We have the elements that are attracted to Elm within us all—if we are truly honest with ourselves instead of trying to hide that which makes us less than perfect.

If we look inside ourselves, there is some form of connection to depression, darkness and misfortune within us (even if this is ancestral) and it is this that connects us to those we encounter with similar traits and draws contractive dynamics towards us. By using Elm, we can shift away from these connections and then soothe with other essences.

Therefore Elm can be used at the beginning of a treatment for those who have constant misfortune and are always having accidents or crises. It is excellent when used in times of severe trauma that appears to be happening 'outside', yet is actually connected to some deeply suppressed part of our psyche.

The Elm Essence is also a wonderful tonic for those who are destined to die young or have terminal illness for Elm reminds us of the greater picture – the energy beyond the physical. For Elm may succumb physically to disease, he may be associated with the aspects of life we would rather deny, yet he lives on and energetically is still sacred and eternal.

CHESTNUT

This essence is a combination of two different viewpoints: The Sweet Chestnut and the Horse Chestnut. The Sweet Chestnut is a stunning tree, with large finger-like leaves and edible nuts in autumn, whilst the Horse Chestnut has beautiful columns of white, pink or red flowers and produces 'conkers'—a favourite of children's games.

This results in three main divisions of this essence, which are: Sweet, White and Red, combining to create harmony and balance together, whilst offering separate influences for those who require it. To use the essence, simply Calibrate using a trigger "***** Chestnut" where ***** is Sweet, Red or White.

Sweet Chestnut works with the nurture of family whatever form the family unit takes. This could be traditional, single parent, partners without children, single person with pets, community, etc. The Sweet Chestnut helps us to assert the energy of our home and family – keeping us free of negative reactions and 'external' influences that may be detrimental.

The essence of Sweet Chestnut helps partnerships and unions, the coming together of people, lives and situations as well as the easing of the evolutionary process, helping couples to learn together and maintain a balance within their union. The essence will also help with areas surrounding abundance, plenty, nourishment and the ability to provide for yourself and your family.

White Chestnut works upon the emotional and cerebral levels of the body, as well as the assimilation of food and digestion. It can yield excellent results when working on the issues of obesity and over-eating, especially when coordinated with some other form of therapy such as NLP or hypnosis.

Red Chestnut focuses on organs such as the liver, kidneys, spleen, etc. It repairs the damage done vibrationally from smoking, drinking, drug-use and other substance abuse while working on mental levels to help ease cravings and addictive tendencies. As with the White, Red Chestnut yields the best results when supported by other therapies.

The theme running through the Chestnut Essence is that of the inconsistencies between the physical and spiritual selves – the over use of material things, food, drugs, etc. and then the blocking of other things such as money, abundance, nurture of the family and so on.

The essence addresses these imbalances, enabling us to fulfil what is lacking in our energy and thus negating the need to use drugs or over-eat, etc. The essence then works on the discordance between the two realms where the limiting beliefs we are giving as children have placed a finite boundary on the amount of energy we 'deserve'.

COPPER BEECH

More Copper Beech have added their views to Celtic Reiki than any other species of tree! These most beautiful trees colour our landscapes with their spectacular display of dark red or purple leaves that sometimes turn a rich coppery-gold.

The Copper Beech Essence is the perspective of source trees from various locations, with contrasting sizes and ages; from old, wise trees that are so big they dominate their surroundings, to the smallest saplings and young trees.

One of these individuals is a weeping Copper Beech that was rescued from a Garden Centre in Cornwall. He had not been watered for long time, was propped up at an angle, and, in the heat of the summer, was dying. He called to the people that walked past him and they were reaching out and touching his last few leaves without realising why.

Copper Beech is a Universal healer, for the Essence of this species contains mostly individuals who have been rescued, cured from disease or have otherwise suffered and survived the trauma to make a full recovery. Hence the essence makes an excellent treatment for recovering from life-threatening trauma and also commonplace disease and life issues. All this, as well as retaining the elements of standard Beech trees, too!

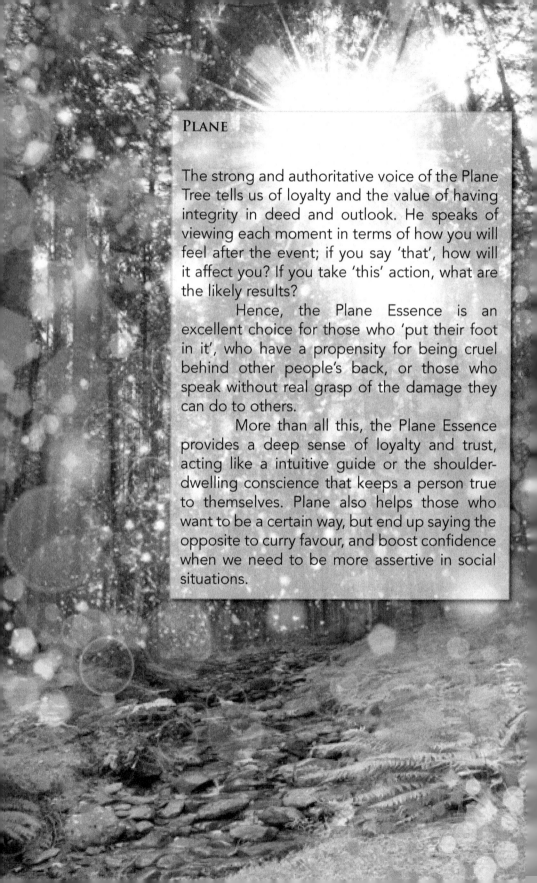

PLANE

The strong and authoritative voice of the Plane Tree tells us of loyalty and the value of having integrity in deed and outlook. He speaks of viewing each moment in terms of how you will feel after the event; if you say 'that', how will it affect you? If you take 'this' action, what are the likely results?

Hence, the Plane Essence is an excellent choice for those who 'put their foot in it', who have a propensity for being cruel behind other people's back, or those who speak without real grasp of the damage they can do to others.

More than all this, the Plane Essence provides a deep sense of loyalty and trust, acting like a intuitive guide or the shoulder-dwelling conscience that keeps a person true to themselves. Plane also helps those who want to be a certain way, but end up saying the opposite to curry favour, and boost confidence when we need to be more assertive in social situations.

Sugar Maple

The essence of the Sugar Maple is both light in sensation and immensely powerful in effect, especially on physical and material levels. It is no surprise that this dynamic essence is excellent when working with results pertaining to money, finances, and material gain or challenge.

Whilst very good at working with the clearing of debt and for bringing in money at times of need, it is recommended that this essence is used pro-actively to obtain genuine abundance, as opposed to the clearing of deficits.

This is done through the manifestation of results and emotional states, rather than 'hard, cold cash'. Explore why you want abundance; what are the experiences you want to have and the emotions you want to feel? Is money the path to achieve these, or is the end result beyond that of money. Focus on real wealth – wealth of mind, emotion, body and spirit, as well as the wealth that is commonly accepted.

On emotional and cerebral layers, the Sugar Maple brings a perspective of laugher and humour, because if Celtic Reiki were a party, the Sugar Maple Essence would be the one, by the bar, telling the jokes and showing people how to have fun!

OLIVE

Wrapped within the folds of the Olive Essence is an ancient wisdom that reminds us that the best way to prolong life is to enjoy life to the full and invest in happiness.

In our modern, information-heavy world, we are often told what to 'take' and what not to do, if we want to stay young and healthy. Very often, however, we become so fixated by the 'rules' and rituals of youth that we forget to live!

When wrinkles appear and those grey hairs start to become more prominent than the hairs-of-colour, do not view this as 'getting old', but more as a privilege – a precious and rare gift that so many do not ever get to experience.

The processes and signs of age are like any other step on our journey—there to be relished and enjoyed. So often, though, we are told that the first thirty years of life are the best and age is not desirable. The Olive Essence readdresses this myth and tells us to enjoy your age, your growth through time and the cycles of your body – you have earned every line through tear and smile.

This time will never come again, so do not wish it away for the memory of a lost youth – enjoy every moment of life, for this in itself will keep you younger and happier than any strange regime or practice of deprivation!

LIME

The perspective of the Lime offers cohesion and synthesis to elements and areas of life, which seem fragmented, separate, or incompatible. And, instead of simply gluing these contrasting regions together, the Lime Essence finds the most conducive way of blending and creating harmony in any union.

When used creatively or inventively, Lime can be seen to work miracles, from healing challenging relationships to fixing broken dreams. On physical levels, the Lime works wonders on speeding the recovery of fractured limbs, spiritually, the Lime helps those who are lost, reconnect to their faith.

Another aspect of the Lime is its ability to create compatibility where two completely conflicting forces come together.

Where many would expect to see sparks, the Lime produces active discussion, diplomacy and compromise in the most valuable sense of the word. Therefore, Lime is not only remarkable at bringing elements together, it also fixes and partners other essences; even if they don't seem to go together upon first inspection.

THE WILD SERVICE TREE

This beautiful tree of crinkled leaf and spiky seed cleanses the heart with a warming, loving perspective. With what can best be described as an embrace, the Wild Service Tree helps shift a person's view of the world to a more loving place, where they see the ways people hurt each other and can understand how to resolve these issues.

The essence gives a more expanded place from which to empower others with wisdom and the notion that we are only responsible for our own lives and our own power, regardless of what we may choose to believe to the contrary!

HORNBEAM

The song of the Hornbeam is a eulogy; a celebration of life when death comes. Yet Hornbeam is not a perspective of sadness or loss; it is a healing of grief, a means to great happiness in the face of such transition and change.

To this end, the Hornbeam is as valuable at times of togetherness, as it is when we must say goodbye to those we love. For the essence enables us to value each other more—to love and be loved.

The Hornbeam Essence offers a legacy after the

ones we love travel onto new adventurers and it also provides us with a positive approach to death. This is not 'strength' or 'courage'; the Hornbeam does not want us to see death as something to be overcome. No, the view of this little tree is very specific.

When we die, no matter what the circumstances or events, we reach a moment where we experience bliss—an overwhelming, all-encompassing love that engulfs us. This very simple fact is not the work of a cold, sterile, and mechanical Universe—it is a very subtle hint that we are all part of a benevolent source.

This amazing and incomprehensible intelligence does not want to see us alone and afraid (we are too proficient in that during our life!), it wants us to know joy. When death of this physical life comes, we spend the last few moments with our physical body, experiencing it find peace and freedom, before remembering who we truly are.

This is not an event that need be feared for ourselves or those we love. The Hornbeam knows this profound wisdom and whispers it to us in many different ways. To heal our grief, comfort our lost and tame our fear; this essence is with us and all we need do is call.

The Mighty Sequoia

The Sequoia is not found naturally in the Celtic areas of Europe, yet its powerful abilities for healing and assisting us energetically meant that I wanted to include this immensely beneficial and remarkable energy in the practice of Celtic Reiki.

Working on the connection between Heaven and Earth, the Sequoia essence offers us the ability to walk between worlds and yet be in all places at once. By doing so, we are able to bring the information of other realms to us here in our everyday lives.

Sequoia is magic and has the ability to manifest

heaven on Earth and helps us to live our own individual perception of Heaven, perfection, bliss, etc. It is the energy of sudden change and rapid evolution and can be used as a tonic whenever a subject is going through times of huge growth, spiritually, emotionally, intellectually or physically.

Hence, Sequoia is excellent for teenagers, whose bodies are changing rapidly, for women in pregnancy or at the menopause or just before, during and after death to help us come to terms with the transition.

THE EUCALYPTUS

Eucalyptus, as with Sequoia, is not native to the Celtic regions, yet it is an incredible healer and invigorator, its fast growth and resilience makes it another excellent candidate for Celtic Reiki practice and usage.

Physically, Eucalyptus has many uses being an analgesic when used with physical pain and excellent for diseases of the respiratory tract, sinuses and head area in general. The essence works well on blockages, so is useful in the treatment of a blocked nose, stuffy head, catarrh on the chest and so on.

Whereas Sequoia works well on periods of fast growth and rapid change, Eucalyptus works on the sluggish and slow, invigorating and stimulating, so is excellent for issues such as ME, lethargy, bad circulation, blocked lymph, mental haze and confusion, aches and so on.

Spiritually, Eucalyptus is very assertive and helps one find one's own strength to stand against strong disruptive energy such as electrical equipment, etc. The essence will nurture and help people to feel safe and secure in whatever they do, offering the sensation of vibrancy and of feeling awake enough to face whatever lies ahead of us on our journey.

THE LITTLE ACACIA TREE

The Little Acacia Tree is a testament to how one so small can be so great in the face of adversity. This adversity comes not only as in shock or trauma, but in the tiny challenges that build slowly, over time. These ever-increasing issues seem like nothing when viewed individually, but gradually they merge together to form long periods of sustained hardship. These are times that Acacia offers strength, endurance and the ability to overcome anything.

Personified by a small, seemingly insignificant tree that copes with unimaginable desert heat, he is waiting for rain that never comes, having to dig deeper and deeper for a few patches of moisture – enough to survive another day. However, there is no sign of complaint or lack of courage, for this tree is happy to be alive and knows that whilst he must dig to survive, the experience is one worth fighting for.

THE TREE OF HEAVEN

The heavenly serenity of this remarkable essence tells of euphoria, joy and an epiphany that by its very definition is beyond words. This tree symbolises every individual that lives to achieve some task or goal with a passion— be it a love of one's work, one's family, one's art, or simply a passion for life.

The Tree of Heaven has a perspective that shifts us to a place where we can perceive the very things and aspects of life that will help us come alive. She wakes us from a deep slumber, our waking trance, and points us in the direction of a new, wide-eyed wonder for what we never knew we loved so much.

Especially useful for people who have lack-lustre lives, those who grind and trudge through a life of drudgery and soul-withering routine; the Tree of Heaven opens the senses to a newfound zest and joy that is never forgotten. When connected to the essence, people literally come alive once again; sparkly and full of energy, they set about striving for their dreams and ambitions once again.

THE MONEY TREE (JADE PLANT)

Traditionally, the 'Money Tree' is seen as a source of financial abundance and wealth, though the Celtic Reiki Essence of Money Tree seems to be connected to 'richness', not only in monetary terms, but of experience and enthusiasm, happiness and love.

Harvested from several individuals, the essence was initially formed of one Money Tree plant; a tiny little plant that was covered in paint and left to die in a box. Rescued, loved, and nurtured, the tree is now quite huge and an absolute picture of health and vitality.

When the leaves of the Money Tree are left on the surface of the soil, they take root and a whole new plant grows. This is represented in the perspective of the Money Tree Essence through the growth and expansion it creates. When triggered in treatment or manifestation, the essence grows exponentially, forming a dynamic where wealth, love, health, joy, or any positive request grows dramatically.

THE LILAC TREE

The sensory delight of the Lilac Tree makes it a lasting favourite amongst gardeners and garden admirers alike! The essence of the Lilac tends to mirror this joy of sensory experience, as it focuses our senses on pleasurable feelings and sensations. Through this process comes a deeper, more profound result – we learn to appreciate the transitory and fleeting moments that are gone, as soon as they arrive.

For often it is those minute glimpses of time that stay with us the longest. A passing glance, a brief encounter, a waft of scent, an exquisite taste, a touch, a glint, a smile; all these things become of value when we understand how important every second is. Thus, the Lilac essence has a way of heightening our senses, keeping our consciousness sharp and ready to soak up every last fragment that drifts in and out of our lives.

THE BUDDLEIA

The Buddleia or 'Butterfly Bush' is extremely similar in look and perspective to the Lilac; and both have the perspective of transitory moments. Yet, whereas the Lilac Essence is of fleeting sensation, the Buddleia Essence enables us to saturate ourselves in the transitory dynamics and situations we encounter.

A wedding day, auspicious event, fond farewell, first date, heartbreaking goodbye, first Christmas, graduation day, the realisation of some goal or achievement – whenever we encounter those times we want to remember, the Buddleia will assist in the crystallisation of experiences.

THE WOODS

THE WALNUT

The essence of the Walnut Tree speaks to us of eternity and the endurance of certain themes. These themes are varied and often contrasting, but are very much a part of the Universe, and in some cases, human nature. The need for connection, for example, is a theme that manifests in different ways for people, from the loving relationship, to the supporting of a team in sports, the patriotic citizen to the quiet and contemplative druid in communion with the Earth. There is a fragile beauty in the way these eternal themes appear to each of us in our own perspective; a beauty that is strengthened in the language of the Walnut.

THE ROSEWOOD

The Rosewood reminds us of contrast in unity, how we often discover similarity in those we view as different from us, whereas people how we feel connected to, often contrast with us in some major way.

This profound message of how different and yet, how identical we are, shows us the interconnected nature of all things and how what we view as separate from us, is actually part of who we are. Therefore we glimpse the source of all things through the perspective of Rosewood; we catch a momentary flash of the self in everything, no matter how different or removed we may feel.

THE TEAK

There is continuity in the essence of the Teak that somehow mirrors the eternity of Walnut and the unity of Rosewood. For the Teak essence whispers to us of how things remain the same; that even at times of total change there is familiarity.

When things appear completely different and unknown, this essence offers comfort in the notion that things have not changed—it is merely our perspective that changes. Just as the sun always rises and sets; we perceive a world constantly shifting and evolving. Though, it is not the sun that tracks across the sky; it is actually the Earth that is moving around the sun!

THE EBONY

This essence is both a mystery and a paradox; it speaks to us of aspirations and the want of achievement, yet invites us to envelop ourselves in the stasis and serenity of being. The Ebony Essence is both expansive and stable; it moves us forward, yet holds us still; in bliss of the place we are in right now. At the heart of this conundrum is the notion of trees that are not ebony, appearing to be ebony—mimics and effigies of a valued truth. Therefore the essence speaks of the aspiration that others experience to become more like you and the realisation that you are the genuine article!

THE ARBUTUS

This elusive and much underused essence has an awe-inspiring wonder wrapped within its perspective. The Arbutus (or Strawberry Tree) Essence personifies a sacred beauty that is very apparent when you know what you are looking for, but is so often missed by the masses. This essence is of the smile that is not reciprocated, the rainbows in dewdrops that businesspeople walk past without noticing, the song that lifts the soul, yet is drowned out by the throng of a crowd. The Arbutus' song brings our forgotten and 'lost' qualities to the surface and lets the world recognise our own, unique gifts.

THE WILD ONES

THE WILD CHERRY

There is a sweetness with the Wild Cherry that washes away regret, bitterness, and hatred that has been bottled up inside and left to rot a person emotional and mentally. Like gazing upon the first blossom of spring and being stopped in one's tracks by the beauty, colour, and vibrancy of these stunning trees, the Wild Cherry Essence stops a person emotionally and in a moment, allows all the trapped pain and stagnancy to dissolve into something new, something better.

THE WILD ROSE

The Wild Rose is soothing and gentle; a perspective that warms and caresses even the weariest of hearts. Its gentle song and light, uplifting energy enable a person to snuggle down, peaceful and serene, to sleep in a refreshing and revitalising slumber. Yet, there is a strength surrounding this essence that is unlike how it feels or acts. This intense power is merely suggested by the results that are achieved by its use in treatment. For the Rose is a guardian, a defender, and friend who will keep you safe with a gentle perfume and soft-hued petal; never letting on about the thorns that keep the outside world at bay!

THE WILD GARLIC

This potent healer cleanses and detoxifies; creating a radical shift in a person's outlook and overall health. Working on all levels of being, the physical and emotional purging that can be created from the use of this essence are astounding.

Cerebrally, the Garlic offers sharpness of mind and innate focus, whilst spiritual growth and letting-go of limitation propel to new layers of awakening. Also excellent for fevers, chills, aches and pains, a sore throat and a headache, the Wild garlic is the essence equivalent of the cure your grandmother used to heal all those little coughs and colds!

THE WILD PRIMROSE

A flash of creamy butter-yellow on a spring morning and the easing of winter's harsh effects; the Wild Primrose symbolises healing and renewal after dark and hostile times. As one of the first flowers to bloom in spring, the essence of this beautiful plant has come to represent that the worst is over and from here on in, the days will get brighter and longer.

This essence is also excellent at times when preparation is needed, planning and the sowing of seeds. For the healing and nurturing of Wild Primrose is focused on the year ahead and what one can best get in shape for the harvest to come.

THE WILD ORCHID

Of vibrant colour and complex shape, the rare Wild Orchid of late spring and summer, tells us of halcyon days and heady reward for past efforts and hardships. The harvest is near and these moments are now to be embraced.

Drink heartily from the stream, taste the sweetness of summer fruits, soak up the richness of each colour and relish every scent. It is a period of wringing every last drop of joy from your life and dancing, singing, revelling in each blessed second we have.

Conversely, this essence is excellent for those in the darkness and bitterest of winters; for the aged and the depressed; anybody who needs a simple reminder of how wonderful things can be when the sun is shining and the birds are singing!

THE POISONS

THE HEMLOCK

The hemlock despite its deadly gaze offers deep-acting, physical treatment for issues of the mid abdomen and throat. There are themes of spiritual awakening, finding one's spiritual path or voice, and the expression of joy that weave through this essence, during treatment. For manifestation purposes, hemlock works well with the achievement of better overall health and well-being.

THE FOXGLOVE

The foxglove gently caresses issues of the heart, both physically in connection to heart dis-eases and emotionally, adding a soft and soothing touch of healing when gripped by the pain of unrequited love. There is an innate beauty about the digitalis' essence that is matched only by its power. The grace that is offered to one's heart and soul through connection to this essence seems boundless and quite magical.

THE MONKSHOOD

The essence of mysteries and secrets, the Monkshood is an enigma of mind and spirit. Use to uncover deception, but also to cloud what is so clear! For, when a well-trodden path no longer gets you where you want to be, you may need to forget what you know with such clarity and discover a new way forward. This essence offer a way of shrouding the habitual and familiar, so that you can dive into the unknown, test your will and create yourself anew.

THE LABURNUM

The bright essence is fizzy and bubbly, rather similar in feel to the Onn perspective. Yet, there are dark secrets here! This essence has many uses for uncovering deception and uncloaking the false, but there is one action of the essence that excels beyond all else—it helps you to uncover deception in those closest to you. Being lied to, or hurt by somebody you trust can be devastating; the Laburnum Essence, will help you see right through the make-believe that is right before your eyes.

THE DEADLY NIGHTSHADE

The silent and the dark; such power and cruelty are contained within the nuances of this essence, however, these do not create reactions that are in themselves negative. An excellent essence for the treatment of depression, especially when the focus of that treatment feels worthless, bullied, or without hope. Perfect for those with notions of suicide or a deep sense of hopelessness— that they are a failure—this perspective draws darkness to itself, thus moving the clouds that block out the sun.

THE SENSUAL ESSENCES

THE POPPY

Of vibrant red, of blood and passion; this essence is a heady mix of exhilaration, excitement and serenity. For whilst its dynamic and powerful perspective offers a motivation force unlike else, there is also a calmness within. Like the runner, who enters a trance-like state whilst she flies like the wind, or the warrior who faces a ferocious battle with quiet dignity; this essence is the space within the fury, the eye of the storm, and peace that calms the most tormented soul.

THE CALICO

The soft, velvety leaves of this plant are mirrored in its perspective of contemplation and relaxation. This truly kinaesthetic essence gives deep insight to those who are confused and enfolds the most troubled mind with clarity of purpose. Yet, this is not a calming essence, for within the profound peace it offers, is a frenetic dance of proactive focus and definite action. For those who feel stuck, or cannot seem to cope with their struggles, Calico presents us with the ability to keep moving, but in a more productive way.

THE NIGHT SCENTED STOCK

The rich and dizzying scent of this most beautiful plant fills the evening air, like an almost tangible wall of aroma. Thick and silky with a sweetness that overwhelms the senses, the Night Scented Stock offers a perspective of centred cohesion to those who feel as if they have come undone. When circumstances feel shattered and fragmented, leaving the subject unable to comprehend everything that is happening, this essence is like spiritual and cerebral glue that fastens everything together, forming a strong resolve for the path ahead.

THE VANILLA ORCHID

There is no flavour quite like that of the vanilla pod—one of the most relished and sought-after tastes (and aromas) known to humankind. The essence of the vanilla orchid is rather like an emotional cleanser, but its action is as soft and gentle as to be almost unnoticed. This is not through weakness or ineffectual behaviour, but through an innate kindness that permeates this most beautiful perspective.

Thus, Vanilla is ideal for those who need emotional cleansing, but literally cannot take any more; those at the end of their tether who could not withstand the rigours of more radical detoxifications.

THE BAMBOO

The essence of sound and hearing, the Bamboo offers ease of communication and prosperity through different parties coming together to talk. This makes the Bamboo Essence excellent for salespeople or negotiators who are striving for success through their communications. Anybody who is looking for achievement through linguistics or telecommunication, or even other forms of transmission, such as music or electronic communication can benefit from Bamboo, whose perspective is traditionally equated with luck and prosperity.

THE ROOTS

THE GINGER ROOT

The Essence of Ginger is fiery and warming; an excellent cleanser that centres primarily on the head, heart, and abdominal regions of the body. The health benefits of the physical root have been known for millennia, however, in perspective-orientated terms, the Ginger Essence is equally influential in matters of physical well-being, stimulating and energising. Emotionally this essence invigorates the emotions and causes mental alertness, an increase in cerebral acuity and improved memory function.

THE GINSENG ROOT

Ginseng, like Ginger, is also a stimulator, although here the foci of physical treatment are the head, circulatory system and sexual regions of the body. The essence can help to increase blood flow, cause arousal and improve energy levels, especially when treating ME or lethargy.

Cerebrally, the essence awakens and helps to alleviate fogginess or sluggishness caused through lack of sleep. The Ginseng Essence is also excellent when cold or caught in icy environments to heat the body, though it is not a substitute for adequate clothing!

THE SARSAPARILLA ROOT

The sweet and subtle Essence of Sarsaparilla is wonderful for helping those who are embittered or have a very contractive view of life. For the ill-tempered, martyr or victim mentality, this root essence grounds in a very positive way, but not so much as to allow the spirit to rise up and become more joyous.

All the root essences are grounding, though this is the least 'earthy' of the perspectives, offering lightness and humour, as well as the ability to laugh.

THE TURMERIC ROOT

The most calming of all the roots, Turmeric is the essence to use when nerves are frayed and tempers are short. Excellent as an overall physical and mental healer, this essence promotes the-healing of wounds, dis-ease and emotional trauma, as well as sharpening the mind, rather like Ginseng and Ginger do.

In fact these three essences create a wonderful trinity where mental sharpness and general brain function need improving, but the stimulating effects of Ginger and Ginseng alone leave the subject feeling nervous or apprehensive.

THE LIQUORICE ROOT

Liquorice Essence is the perspective of harmony, balance and centred focus. Working well on the digestive system, it regulates the processing of food and is brilliant for helping ease both constipation and diarrhoea, because of its balancing effects.

The Essence of Liquorice is also wonderfully suited to assisting and supporting people with confidence issues and those of a shy disposition, especially when the subject suggests that they find it difficult to think of what to say in social situations, or they hold back in saying what they want to say, until it is too late.

THE
WOODLAND
OR
ELVEN
ESSENCES

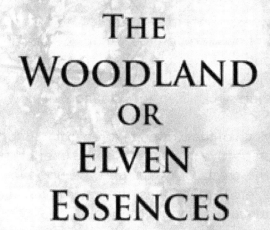

BRIGHID [BRIG-HEED]

The Goddess Brighid is one of the deities whose reputation flows through the various Celtic communities, from Ireland and Western Britain to Continental Europe. Her essence is of the light and fire; she is a healer and mother that symbolises the creation of new things or states.

Much of the written text regarding Brighid tells of higher perspective in a physical sense (mountain summits, hilltops, the crests of waves and the uppermost part of any flame, etc.), mention is often also given in respect of cerebral functions of higher thought and wisdom.

Essentially, in a Celtic Reiki context, the Brighid Essence could be perceived as creation from inspiration to completion. As the poet journeys from spark to sonnet and the blacksmith from raw metal to shoe or sword, Brighid is the guiding light and voice that beckons. She helps us heal in times of dis-ease and offers the comfort of a mother to her child when frightened or in pain.

RHIANNON [REE-AN-NON]

Welsh mythology describes Rhiannon as a queen who is wrongly accused of a terrible crime (killing her child) and eventually vindicated. Whilst there is little mention of her goddess status in historical texts, the modern perspective of Rhiannon often equates her with the Goddess of Horse, Epona, and with integral associations with the Moon.

The Celtic Reiki perspective of Rhiannon focuses on the passage of wrongful accusation and eventual restoration. This essence helps all those who have been lied about, accused of something they have not done, or found themselves in a situation where others assumed the worst.

Where one is subject to an awful injustice or a complex situation that others interpret as something other than what it is, Rhiannon helps bring truth to the surface of the situation.

The paradoxical thread of this perspective is that often, both or all parties feel slighted in circumstances that involve accusation, so be prepared for a sharp awakening if Rhiannon presents you with the responsibilities you personally hold in the dynamic that has been created.

TARANIS [TA-RA-NIS]

The foundations of the god, Taranis, are believed to originate with the Roman god Jupiter and bear remarkable parallels with Thor, the Norse god. As the deity of thunder, there are many connections to cleansing and renewal through the Celtic Reiki Essence.

Just as the god himself was viewed as having the dual nature of joy and good-humour, combined with fury and punishment, the essence is the perspective of detoxification and rebirth. The detoxification can be painful and cleansing frequently asking us to confront the aspects of our psyche that we would rather bury and forget. However, rebirth is an experience of great joy and wonderment.

When using the essence of Taranis, the emphasis is always on rebirth and the exhilaration of some new, expanded state of being. Just as Taranis was slow to anger, the cleansing properties of this essence are rarely seen. Yet, be aware that when they come, they come with the fury of the thunderstorm!

CERRIDWEN [KAR-HID-WHEN]

In the modern perspective of Celtic philosophy and spirituality, the Goddesses have become interchangeable in perspective, with common themes being the moon, inspiration, and poetry! With academic texts focusing on the Celtic mythology in a textual sense (as opposed to a spiritual sense) and web texts equating each goddess with the same attributes, we look to oral traditions to gain a clearer idea of who is who.

Cerridwen is often viewed as symbolic of the Earth and the natural world, as well as being what some call, Goddess of the Underworld.

To maintain the relevance of Celtic Reiki in a modern world, we tend to avoid such 'boxy' terms that pertain to good, bad, black, white, etc. Thus, one perspective of Cerridwen is of contraction into the physical and expansion into what exists beyond the physical.

In the philosophy of some higher force, contracting into the physical world for the purpose of experience and the physical expanding back toward Source when the purpose is fulfilled, we see a definite dynamic emerging. This dynamic not only encompasses a person's life, but of all physical things, including situations, thoughts, moments of time, and so on.

Everything that exists in the physical world has a purpose, it is Source contracted. Once the purpose has been experienced, source expands back out of being. This is the essence of Cerridwen – manifestation of the divine in the physical and the physical experiencing the divine through time and space.

LLEU [CLUE]

The mythos of Lleu was bathed in trickery, deceit, mystery and a curse that would be the core of this deity's story. The God of Light, Lleu brings an essence of potentially powerful force to Celtic Reiki.

The concept of being deceived, treachery, hidden challenges and being the focus of another's ill-will form the dis-ease that the Lleu Essence repatterns with light and expansion into bliss.

The essence symbolises freedom from pain and the hurts that we feel because of the actions of others. However, the real strength of this essence is the realisation that it was our own actions that led us towards the pain—we are only hurt by others, when we give them permission to do so.

Just as Lleu empowered others to take his life, we give our own personal power to others through blame and the refusal to take responsibility for our own actions. Yet through his actions, Lleu was set free and became more than he could ever be in physical form.

SILVANUS [SIL-VEY-NOUS]

The origin of Silvanus is Roman, as opposed to Celtic, yet there are definite parallels between Silvanus and Cernunnos; the Horned God of the woodland. These similar perspectives offer us a valuable experience in the discovery of similar, yet contrasting essences.

Silvanus, also a woodland deity, forms the essence of the woodland Realm, yet of a more physical perspective than that of the Master Essence, Cernunnos.

Silvanus is, in many ways, closer to the human perspective, as he is connected to pastures and the use of forstry for human needs. The keeping of livestock and use of the natural world for food, etc. are all the domain of Silvanus.

As the only Roman deity of the Celtic Reiki Woodland Essences, he also represents the power of empire and how the physical (human) world often dominates the natural world. Yet through working with the Silvanus Essence, we can learn how to Master our own sense of ownership and possession toward the Cernunnos Mastery Essence that is derived through experience, as opposed to Orientation.

THE
ELEMENTAL
ESSENCES

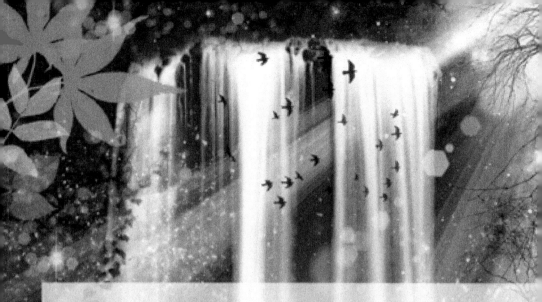

Bearn—Space—[Bi-een]

Bearn is the first of five elemental essences in Celtic Reiki that encompasses the elements of our world and thus, connecting us to different aspects of the Celtic Reiki Essences. So, for example, if you wish to create a more grounded effect in your treatment, Pridd (Earth) Essence will create a more physical connection. On the other hand, if you wanted a lighter effect, you might use Annal (Air) in your treatment forest.

'Space' creates a void – a place where energy in non-reactive and therefore neutral. This would feel like there is no energy wherever Bearn flows, yet we know that energy is everywhere and infinite, so Bearn simply halts our reaction with energy.

This makes Bearn Essence the first choice when working with subjects who have connected into something that is either sapping their energy or creating massive energetic reactions. For instance, somebody may be following a dream that is not on their path and therefore projecting energy to a place that they will never reach or possibly they have connected into something very angry and are channelling an anger that is not their own.

If at any time your subject is connected to something that is harming or draining them, Bearn can be directed at the source of damage (as opposed to directed at the subject) and will disconnect your subject from their focus by making it neutral to them.

Pridd—Earth—[preed-th]

The Pridd Essence grounds the connection to the treatment, bringing it more into the physical, creating deeper clearings and more integral change. Essential whenever a subject reacts to treatments in a strong way with many effects during the treatment but little or no improvement afterwards. Using Pridd will create a very material and physical connection, bringing the effects of each Tree Vibration to earth where it can produce stronger detoxification and a much greater healing effect or faster and more direct manifestation of goals.

TAN—FIRE—[TAN]

The Tan Essence adds vibrancy to any treatment and thus creates a viewpoint that is energised. Tan is stimulating, and enables treatments that have a soporific effect to become revitalising while still retaining their relaxation qualities. Remember that fire burns wood, so you may find the actual Tree Essences lose some of their individual characteristics in place of the energetic power, yet this is often better than creating a treatment that pushes a person too far from alertness and awareness.

DWR—WATER—[DAU-R]

Dwr offers a smoother flow of energy vibrations, especially on the emotional and mental levels where blockages can prevent treatment. The fluidity of Dwr makes it a wonderful candidate when fashioning a treatment that envelops your subject and washes through them, invigorating, yet cleansing and calming. Adding the Dwr Essence to your treatment will enable you to create 'mood' and atmosphere in the subtle changes it makes to the other Tree Essences used. Additionally, in contrast to the dominating qualities of Fire, the Dwr Essence enhances the tree vibrations, as opposed to limiting them.

ANNAL—AIR—[ANN-ARL]

The Essence of the Air: Annal uplifts all connections to the Celtic Reiki vibrations offering a lighter and more expansive feel to the treatment. Valuable in subjects who are tense, closed, physically orientated to the point of being stuck, those who are too focussed on 'stuff' or who are having difficulty in being without doing – i.e.: cannot mediate, relax—do nothing and just 'be'. Annal is like applying a treatment with a feather, it is always soft and gentle, lightening the effects of the clearing and providing therapy that is embracing as opposed to cleansing (you can also use Annal as the wind to clear and nurture into movement).

The
Master Essences
of the
Woodland Realm

THE CELTIC TREE MASTER-PRACTITIONER ESSENCE

KOAD – THE GROVE

CH – [CODE – COY-D – CO-ED]

Koad is the essence of sacred sanctuary; of finding a place within that is not only calm and peaceful, but will enable one to cope if everything seems to be falling apart. The perspective of Koad is surrounding, nurturing, and offers a real sense of security while healing.

Koad can be used in treatment to envelop and assert the client; its nature is to give peace and stillness of mind – to laugh in the face of adversity. It can also be used when other perspectives are not achieving the results one might have hoped for, because of some limiting belief or emotional patterning—it will assist the client in shifting to other essences, moving them beyond habitual behaviour. This tends to increase over a period of time.

Many groves create the perspective of Koad, however the main view of this essence is comprised from an ancient Rowan Grove on Bodmin Moor. This small but ancient place contains Rowan, Oak, Elder, Hazel, Gorse and many other types of tree—all of which are contained in this essence.

We could say that Koad Essence is a symbiotic range of views – one created from many individuals, each contributing a special part of the overall, grove perspective. There are Celtic trees here, as well as other varieties, and whilst these are already contained in the Celtic Reiki Mastery, this cooperative perspective is different: a tree reacts differently on a one-to-one basis than it does in a group.

Koad is the essence of group dynamics and, thus, can be used on large groups of people or wherever teamwork or team spirit is needed. It can also be used to heal disconnected families.

Within the contrasting views of many, comes a unifying dynamic that provides assertion, safety and refuge, where a person can meditate and reflect on their life, their purpose and their mission. Koad is an essence that embraces and in which you can lose yourself for a while.

Physical: Koad works wonders on the nervous system and can have an effect on everything from mild-stress to major nervous disorders. It can be used for Raynaud's Syndrome, numbness, paralysis or palsy. It can also work with hyperactivity, or lethargy, and anywhere where there is too much or too little of something (hyper/hypoglycaemia, hypo/hypertension, etc.).

Emotional/Mental: An overactive mind or imagination. Too much internal monologue – no peace and quiet. Helps a person to remain calm and still even when all around them is falling apart. Introspection (lack of, or too much of).

Spiritual: A spiritual sanctuary, a place of being in the moment.

THE CELTIC TREE MASTER ESSENCE

UNHEWN DOLMEN ARCH

THE NAMELESS TREE (BLANK OGHAM)

[UN-OW-EN DOLL-MAN ARK]

The perspective of the Nameless Tree could best be described as somewhat 'alien', as it is unlike any other tree, plant or living thing. Revered by the Celts, Mistletoe has a rather different connotation in the modern world, for it is parasitic and relies on the host tree for all its nutrients.

If the spread of Mistletoe on a single tree becomes too much, it will eventually kill the host tree. In so many ways, there is a comparison between the Nameless Tree and some of the most feared dis-eases of humankind, such as cancer or HIV/AIDS. And, whilst the Nameless Tree is still seen as sacred in the druidic beliefs, many people find it hard to reconcile the actions of this plant with their own innate love of our tree friends.

The Mistletoe is also known as the 'All Heal', because of its healing properties when healing dis-eases of many a different type and prognosis—and it does so with seemingly miraculous results. It is this innate benevolence and its effect on people (and trees) who really understand the nature of Mistletoe that begs our reconsideration of this much-maligned plant.

For the Mistletoe has many secrets and is blessed by nature. So profound is the wisdom and perspective of the Nameless Tree, that even the most noble trees will become quiet in awe at the thought of it. This is because, on physical layers the Mistletoe only takes; there is no reciprocation, no exchange. However when we investigate what occurs on the cerebral and spiritual layers of the host tree's awareness, we begin to realise that a tree bearing the Mistletoe transcends the physical world. The Nameless Tree provides what could be called a hyperreality that extends beyond the physical and into the realms of utter perfection.

This is mirrored in the Master Essence of the Celtic Trees; The Unhewn Dolman Arch or 'blank ogham'.

Here the All Heal offers us the same transcendence and hyperreality that it imbues its hosts with; an expansion beyond the world of solid things and into a place of delight and knowing.

The Unhewn Dolman Arch has the potential to heal any dis-ease or to act on any level of being in the truest sense of holism that we can imagine. Here there are not symptoms, no discrimination or division; only oneness and the healing of the whole. The essence of the Mistletoe will also help us to understand that what we have been taught to regard as the 'self' is not actually the self at all, but an illusion of limited definition. When we grasp this engrained contraction of parameter that is given to us by our own loved-ones and teachers, it becomes clear that it is not the Mistletoe that kills, it is our own belief of what life is that causes it to 'end'.

There are two distinct perspectives of Mistletoe in Celtic Reiki Mastery; the female and the male. These are usually experienced as two totally different essences, however they are very much part of the same species and viewpoint. The female is more physical, with a greater connection to the Earth—she cares and nurtures what we have and heals what dis-eases us in the present moment of experience. The male is completely alien, seeming unearthly and strange at first, but absolutely and blissfully overwhelming when you let him in. Here is the striver, the pioneer, the seeker and the accumulator. His gaze is always facing towards the future and what is yet to come, what could be, and what we need to do now to achieve it.

Between the two genders, the Unhewn Dolman Arch Essence is the foundation of any Master treatment or practice, including the Orientation processes, Ki Classroom, etc. It also adds a greater degree of expansion to all treatments and therefore must be used with forethought: those who are entrenched in old views and the physical consequences of any action will often block this essence or actively work against its influence. In these cases, it is best avoided until the person can transcend their own limitations.

THE NON-CELTIC TREE MASTER ESSENCE

THE BURNING BUSH

Like the Unhewn Dolman Arch, the Burning Bush is a powerful and somewhat overwhelming tree. There is an aspect of forcefulness about this essence that seems to rip dis-ease from the body and knock one out of conscious awareness. Without introduction or pleasantry, the Burning Bush is a power unlike any other. Even though Celtic Reiki tends to move away from many of the dogmatic traditions of humankind, if ever we come close to the concept of an all-powerful 'Old Testament God', this would be His perspective!

In actuality, the Burning Bush is incredibly benevolent and loving in motivation; it is just the action that is a little brutal! This awe-inspiring love saturates the Orientation to the Non-Celtic Tree Essences and flows, like a stream, through many other aspects of the Celtic Reiki Realms. The harsher abruptness tends to come through in treatment and then is marked only when the client is ready for a major transition on all levels.

Often, after many years of treatment or spiritual work, we reach an understanding that, sometimes, pain is involved in the healing process. As we make tough decisions or reconnect to past pain and move beyond its limiting boundaries, we briefly experience the horror and trauma once again. For many this is too much and they simply contract back into the place where the pain is there, but is not directly affecting them. The Burning Bush, on the other hand, is akin to ripping a plaster away from the skin at great speed; it hurts, but only for an instant.

When one is of an understanding that pain, trauma, and emotional upset can be faced and conquered, we are ready for the Burning Bush, who will pluck out hurt and yank away trauma until your heart's content! Of course, if you intuitively feel that somebody who may not relish the idea of this essence's methodology would also benefit greatly from it, you can combine with an essence that distracts with pleasurable experience or anaesthesia; Saille or Copper Beech, for instance.

THE ELVEN ESSENCE MASTER

CERNUNNOS – THE HORNED ONE

[KERR-N-WHO-NOSS]

As the most powerful and unusual essence of the Woodland Realm, Cernunnos is unique in many ways. The most obvious of these is that this essence is not included in any Orientation of Celtic Reiki. The Cernunnos Essence is learnt through experience and use of the Silvanus Essence. For mastery comes, not with the teachings of others, but through the actions of oneself.

Silvanus, the Roman god of the woodland and natural world, is the perspective of human superiority over the world. It is a perspective that we all have by birthright and encompasses our journey back to nature. This always comes with the belief that we are connected to Earth as humans. Gradually we transcend this view and create a different perspective that is beyond the words of human creation.

As we become less distinct from the Earth and all things of the Earth, we move closer towards the Cernunnos perspective.

For some people this may take weeks, for others years; the important point here is that when you eventually Calibrate to the Cernunnos Essence, you will know it with every fibre of your being! The essence is unmistakable and profound in ways that are unlike any other experience.

Do be aware that some people experience their 'usual' meditation visuals or a voice and assume this is the Cernunnos essence. This is all part of the process, because Calibration is self-regulating… the very fact that you are experiencing such things, hints that you are still viewing from a human perspective.

It is not until you lose who you believe yourself to be and transcend your individual perspective that you become Cernunnos and the Master Essence of the Elven (Woodland) Realm. This is both shocking and exhilarating in ways that cannot be described with words!

The Elemental &

Oceanic Realm Master Essence

Mor – Ocean

[M-hore]

Since the earliest origination of the Celtic Reiki system, there has been extensive inclusion of the worlds oceans, from the Pacific to the Atlantic. The perspective of More expands across the world and transcends the limitations of human, geographical and political borders, making this essence all-encompassing.

The Sea holds a profound truth – what could be viewed as the inner depths of knowledge and wisdom. We spend much of our lives on the surface of a rough ocean, letting life take us on its waves without having any say in the direction we want to head in. The More Essence allows us sink down into the still depths of the sea where we can travel through life with ease and calmness.

Mor is a contrasting view of both unknown wisdom and everything that a person can know. It allows one, with regular use, to learn on all layers of perception: spiritually, mentally, emotionally and physically. The Ocean guides us, showing sacred places and themes that we never knew existed.

Mor is also focused upon travel and can help those with fear of travel, flying, water, etc. In fact, the way this essence perceives human fears, creates profound use in any scenario where a person is frighten or held back through fear. This could be fear of a new venture, fear of some perceived outcome, a phobia, or even fears that manifest as some other emotion or action.

The Mor Essence has a close affinity with all the Oceanic Essences, being the Master Essence of the Furthest Ocean. It also shares a connection to Dwr.

THE
STANDING
STONES

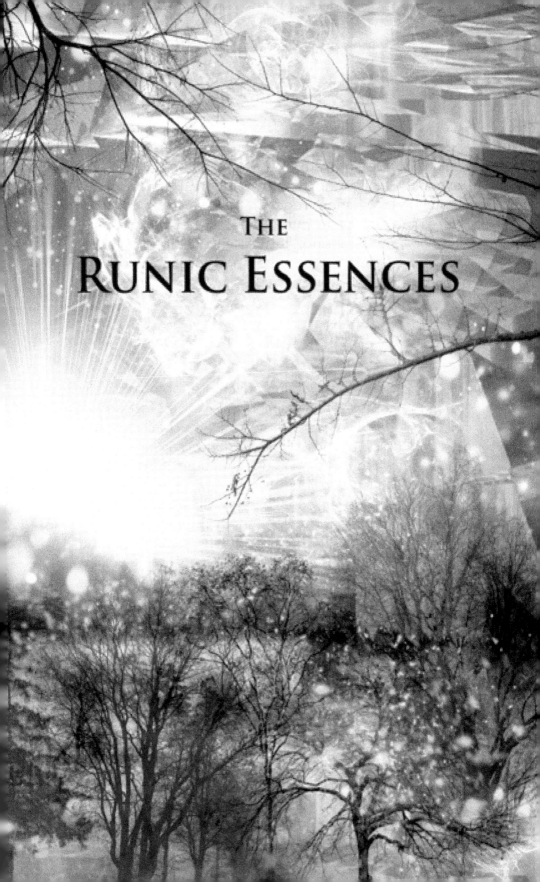

THE
RUNIC ESSENCES

THURISAZ—TH—GIANT—(THOR-EYE-SAYS)

The essence of Thurisaz or 'Thorn' is that of guardianship and the instinctual need to defend. At times of conflict and hatred, when we are offered the opportunity to grow beyond the malice and torment of others, Thurisaz creates a catalyst for change, regeneration and detoxification. Here is the chance to purge the past trauma and pain; cathartic and cleansing, this essence helps us find a new way forward, beyond the need for protection in a physically focused world.

RAIDO—R – CHARIOT – (RYE-THOUGH)

The perspective of travel and adventure, both physically and in the context of life path. The Essence of Raido not only supports travellers and migrants, it actually initiates new and epic voyages of body, mind, and spirituality. Wonderful when used in various situations, from moving house to challenging journeys, a new life to a change of ideals. Whenever one changes direction or focus, the Raido Essence can help smooth the way and when we find ourselves with the opportunity to move beyond stasis and rigidity, this essence can help us find flexibility, transition and expansion. Raido is also an excellent choice when facing injustice – particularly in cases when there has been a perversion of 'natural lore'.

KENAZ—K—TORCH—(KAI-NAYS)

When deluded by hope and at times when we hold out to be 'rescued' or 'saved' by another; be it a partner or some 'mystery gallant knight of trusty steed', the Essence of Kenaz helps us to cut through illusion and reclaim the personal power we so often give away. Transformative, regenerative and inspirational, this essence helps us to harness our own abilities for self-empowerment. Strategic and creative in its dynamics, the Kenaz Essence offers vision, beyond that of the limited physical layers of perception and higher knowledge that is usually beyond our reach.

GYFU—GY—GIFT—(YEE-BOW)

A powerful essence in times of loneliness and co-dependence, when a person places their own happiness in the perspective of another. Martyrs, victims, and those who over-commit themselves can find many hidden treasures in this essence that helps enhance relationships in a balanced way. Generosity and giving are both an integral part of Gyfu, but not in the way of personal sacrifice or lack – this is joyful giving that is done without lack in any way. The Gyfu Essence is particular apt when signing contracts or negotiating deals that involve two parties contributing to some deal or project; ensuring that both are equally rewarded for their part.

WUNJO—W – JOY – (WOON-YO)

Wrapped in the warm folds of joy and comfort, the Wunjo Essence is ecstasy and glory, simply for the sake of pleasure. Wonderful in the creation of personal and spiritual success, the Essence of Wunjo is excellent at helping us move beyond the old view of happiness being a state that needs to be restricted or limited. The traditional worldview of 'life is hard' or joy needing to be restrained for fear of excess are transcended in this perspective. Thus we realise that infinite bliss is possible, without any repercussion or retribution, because we were all born to live as sparks of some higher source of joy.

Peordh—P—Mystery—(Pie-orv)

Secrets and mysteries, the vague and enigmatic, are all brought to the surface by the Essence of Peordh. The perspective of ritual and initiation, this essence is mastery and prophesy, as it unveils what we have not previously recognised. The lifting of the veil and finding one's life purpose are also at the core of this perspective. In therapy practice, Peordh is very helpful in clearing addiction and habitual behaviour.

Eoh- EO – Yew—(eye-o)

The perspective of Eoh is trust and reliability, not in a steadfast and static respect, but in a powerful drive and expansive force. Therefore, the Essence of Eoh is excellent at helping us achieve goals and creating success in the ways we want most. Therapeutically useful for boosting energy levels and alleviating lethargy, Eoh also helps motivation and getting us through the initial stages of any new beginning.

EOLH—X—ELK-SEDGE—(EYE-YE)

Assertion against contractive influences and guardianship are qualities of Eolh. When things appear bigger than oneself, unmanageable, or out of control, this essence can provide stability in turbulent waters. Providing connection to higher levels of wisdom and power, the Essence of Eolh enables us to expand beyond what frightens us, turning the need for protection into a matter of assertion against equals.

HAEGL—H—HAIL – (HAW-GAW)

The Haegl Essence is the perspective of taming the untameable. When the unconscious mind is out of control, destructive and contractive in the results it achieves, Haegl helps the conscious mind bring order and harmony to this primal force. An essence of completion and endings, Haegl invites us to remember that pure force and potential needs direction and without it, can become out-of-control. We all have this same power within, taming it is the task each of us commits to when we shift to the Haegl perspective.

SIGEL—S—SUN—(SEE-JEL)

The force of overwhelming success, victory and vitality are an essential part of this perspective. As we shift from stagnation to flow, regret to faith, pity to honour, the Essence of Sigel is with us. Supporting oneness of all things, including oneself, this essence helps heal fragmental parts of the self and provides us with a more holistic attitude to life. There is a sense of fire (cleansing and motivating) with this essence of life-force and healthy vitality. When in the perspective of Sigel, some might say you have 'inner-fire'.

TIR—T—TYR—(TEA-R)

The perspective of leadership and authority are both highlighted in the Tir Essence, but not in a domineering and governmental way; this is natural charisma and the born leader who others follow instinctively, through choice. Success in legal matters and in competitions also fall under the gaze of the Tir perspective. Knowing oneself and one's goals, inasmuch as being clear-sighted and forthright are the way of the Essence of Tir.

BEORC—B—BIRCH—(BEE-ORK)

Similar to Beh in the Woodland realm, this essence symbolises birth and new beginning. Both essences have, at their hearts, the success of new ventures, the birth of life or some new project, initiation, and the power of the spring. As part of the Standing Stones, this essence has a slight slant towards liberation and the rebirth of oneself as a free and unlimited being.

EH—E – HORSE—(AY-R)

Movement, expansion and change for the better are all of the essence, Eh, though rather than rapid achievement or overnight success, the perspective of Eh comes through long-term progression and clear strategy. Here the gradual development comes with a great sense of achievement and in many cases teamwork. The essence of 'perfection', Eh creates the ideal situation and circumstances, presents us with the right people and conditions and ensures stamina and willpower on the road ahead.

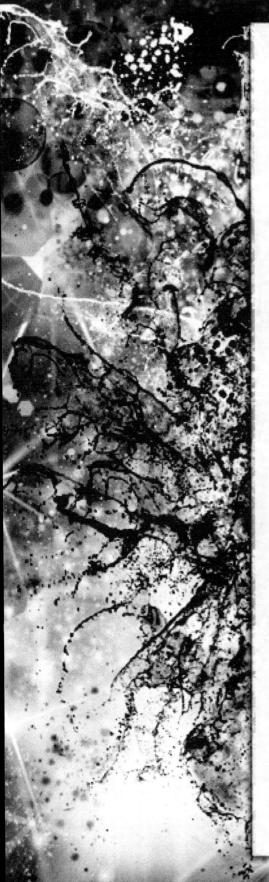

MANN—M—MAN—(MAWN)

The sense of individuality in union, or what some may call 'self-awareness' is the key of Mann. In a vast, interconnected and very complex Universe, the Mann Essence offers simplicity and pure understanding. The perspective of this essence is skilful artistry that conveys much in very little. Also an excellent essence for creating harmony amongst groups and smoothing contention during discussions.

LAGU—L—LAKE—(LAW-GOR)

Fertility and renewal, Lagu is akin to the water, the sea, the motion of fluidity. A deeply healing essence, Lagu provides organic growth, physically and metaphorically – the process of structure evolving gradually and steadily from some foundation or root. The understanding of dreams and hidden depths also weave their way into this perspective, which is similar to Dwr in the Woodland Realm and would also not look out of place in the Further Ocean realm.

NAUTHIZ - N - NEED - (NOW-THESE)

The Essence of Nauthiz helps us to think innovatively in times when challenges seem unsolvable. When confused or perplexed by some seemingly impossible task or situation, Nauthiz offers lateral thinking, creativity, and inspiration to change our viewpoint. With a little bit of patience and a sense of endurance, this essence can work miracles; allowing us to reach for the skies in novel and rather unusual ways!

ISA - I – ICE - (EE-SAW)

The Isa Essence eases frustration and assists us at times when we cannot seem to grasp a particular task or answer. When faced with mental-blocks or inertia in any aspect of life, Isa helps dissipate confusion and lack of mental acuity. The Essence of Isa also nurtures a transcendence of ego, especially in group situations, as well as helping groups to 'gel' cohesively when working together on a project or challenge.

JERA – J - YEAR - (YARE-AWE)

The essence of the harvest, when the effort and commitment to some outcome are achieved with plentiful results and great reward; this is the nature of Jera. Offering the dynamic of momentum and vibrancy, Jera tells us to keep moving forward, building and growing, because success will come eventually. At the core of the Jera perspective is the idea that anybody can achieve their dreams, providing they keep working towards them – the only reason not to attain one's goals is the commitment to not achieving them!

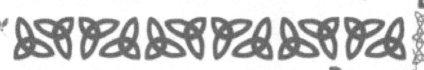

Fehu - F - Wealth - (FAY-WHO)

The Essence of Fehu has the greatest action in areas of material gain and possession. This 'lucky' essence nurtures abundance and financial freedom, so is often associated with success and happiness. In the Nordic perspective, Fehu is held in high esteem for obvious reasons, though it can also be used when social matters are highlighted, for vitality, energy and at times of creation. When we are presented with the opportunity to grow through poverty, loss, or feeling powerless in some challenging situation, Fehu can help us to transcend the current situation and achieve success anew. Fehu boosts self-esteem, focuses the mind and helps us to find the courage within when most needed.

Uruz - U - Wild Ox – (OO-ROCKS)

The Uruz Essence invites us to view life from an attitude of physical strength, speed and wild potential. With the increased physical energy and vitality that we are offered through connection to Uruz, one may feel completely free of limitation; tenacious and bold in action. The influence of this essence can create feelings of being unstoppable, charismatic and powerful, yet when dominated, bullied and feeling weak, Uruz enables us to tap into that deep infinite well of inner-strength and unleash our true spark of independence and leadership.

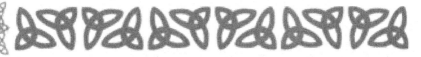

ING—NG—ING—(ENG)

The perspective of the Earth (or Earth God), Ing symbolises internal growth, be it of the individual or of the family, group, or community. Simple pleasures and peaceful days, spent under the warm sunlight of a summer's day, the time of rest after a harvest and all the day's work has been completed. This essence is the absolute must for tying-up loose ends and completing projects. When you have achieved success and all is well, the Ing Essence helps you sleep soundly and take a breath before the next journey begins.

DAEG—D—DAY—(THAW)

When one has hit the wall and suddenly feels as if it is impossible to carry-on, the Essence of Daeg provides a breakthrough; renewed resolve and the conviction of will. This is not only in the sense of some physical trial, but of emotional, cerebral and spiritual tasks as well. Creating the ability to master one's own destiny through will and perseverance, Daeg offers hope and happiness to those who are floundering, certainty to the unsure, and sight to those who have lost their way.

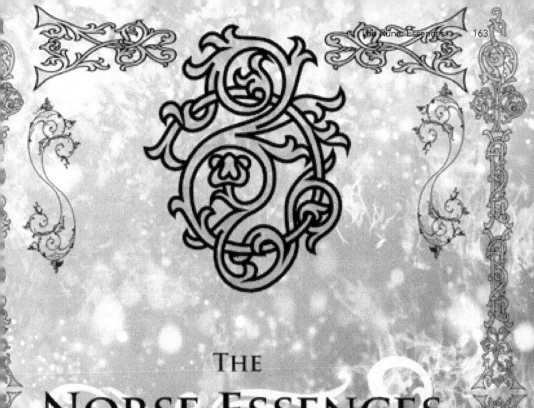

THE
NORSE ESSENCES

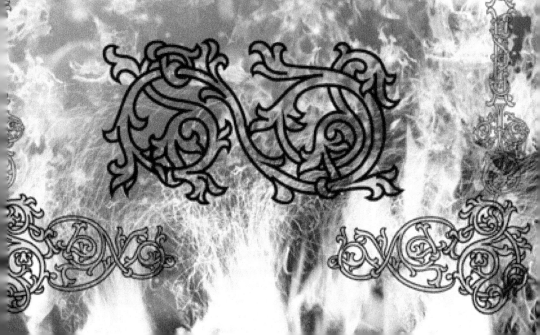

BRAGI [BRA-HAY]

The Norse god of writing and poetry, Bragi is the constant guide and companion of those who express themselves with words. Yet, through use of the Bragi Essence, we learn to transcend words in the expression of our deepest and most heartfelt truth. The son of Odin, Bragi, represents the nature of storytelling and of poetry. The Bragi perspective is peaceful and focuses on the use of words to inspire the spirit, rouse emotions, and create peace through diplomacy and rhetoric, rather than fighting.

There are connections between the Bragi, natural lore and elven realms, thus his essence enriches those of the Woodland Realm. With additional connections between the Bragi Essence and the runic characters of Norse writing, the Runic Essences are also empowered greatly through a shift to the Bragi perspective.

Whenever you require the power of a master orator, diplomat, or negotiator, Bragi will improve the flow and power of the words you use. He creates peace and harmony; he will also help you perfect your persuasive language to help others release their limiting beliefs and progress towards a success-orientated way of behaving.

NJORD [NORD]

The Master of the Ocean and of the Wind, Njord could conjure up the fiercest of storms or the calmest sea. A benevolent and generous deity, His essence is that of compassion and giving, as well as the powerful forces of Earth; those that drive storms and cause crops to germinate.

The father of Freja, his perspective brings abundance and extreme forces to play, yet his is a viewpoint of comparison and contrast. He enables us to see when we are making do, because what we have now is better than what we had previously. In other words, if you are in a situation where life is not fulfilling, or crammed with love and joy, or overflowing with prosperity, yet one is making do with this, because this life is better than the past and trauma of the past, Njord will bring the insight of comparison into your awareness. Suddenly you will begin to see how things could be' the Njord Essence will support you in creating a new reality where you have attained happiness, rather than 'getting by'. This perspective is of awareness, achievement and attainment. It enables one to identify one's needs and to fulfil those needs.

BALDUR [BAAL-DOO-R]

The essence of Baldur, like the god, is of light and happiness. The father of Forseti, he was viewed as a lord or leader; honourable, kind and courageous, his essence is associated with death—not only of the physical body, but any circumstances where the ending of some valued situation or loved relationship is apparent.

The Baldur Essence brings acceptance in a loving and expansive way—by helping us to see the light in any transition. The idea of travelling towards the light, after death, could be used here in a metaphorical way, as we shift to the Baldur viewpoint and see the greater perfection in every loss, transition, or rebirth.

Many believe the world to be cruel, harsh, and a battle for survival—in this world life is cheap and expendable if it means the survival of an idea or particular way of thinking. Baldur helps us to understand the processes of ageing and dying are neither cruel nor harsh—they are deeply private and joyous moments when we get to experience every step of the process.

Each wrinkle or grey hair in the Baldur perspective is a gift of life and conscious experience. He enables us to see beyond death, to the benevolence that guides us each and every step of the way.

FORSETI (FOUR-SET-HEY)

A master of justice and bringer of hope, the perspective of Forseti is like the silver or gold fringe that encompasses a dark storm cloud; a reminder that, even in the darkest and most violent of storms, the sun is still shining and that her glorious light will be seen again.

This is a particularly useful perspective when a person is experiencing legal issues; specifically those that derive from personal justice or natural lore. When one has been treated unfairly, experienced prejudice, slander, libel, or has had something taken from them erroneously, Forseti will help to bring a satisfactory outcome—if a person believes they deserve it and also acts without malice or hatred for the other party.

Forseti Essence is the ability to look deep into the heart of another and see the truth that exists there, whatever that truth may be. It brings our deepest motivations to the surface and guides us towards the essential balance that flows through all things.

Freja [FRAY-YAH]

The Norse goddess of love and beauty, her perspective is from an all-encompassing sense of compassion, devotion and joy that transcends the physical world. Yet Freja is of the love that transcends death, creates life, and motivates terrible wars. She embraces those who have been scarred by horrific trauma and brings healing and comfort to those who thought they could never experience joy again (or do not know what joy is).

The essence of Freja works wonderfully with the Standing Stones essence of Gold and the Oceanic Red Essence. Her perspective is utter compassion, without judgement or condition—she offers a selflessness that takes complete responsibility to uphold and trust in.

Her viewpoint releases blame and enables us to completely turnabout in attitude, circumstance and result. Even when we are faced with old battles, age-old arguments, or deep-rooted pain that we feel others have caused us, Freja can love us so completely, eternally and infinitely, that the wars we hold on to simply fade away into memory.

There are deep connections between Freja and

Frigg, which can be sensed in their essences, yet Freja's perspective is more of universal love, death, and those who are crippled through battle; whatever the context of that battle.

By working with Frigg, we may move bravely, into and beyond the tribulations or trauma we face. By doing so, we travel towards the place where we meet Freja and can heal any wounds we have acquired. This bestows upon us the wisdom we require to achieve what we want to achieve; that wisdom can never be bought, learnt, or obtained in any other way.

SKADI [SCAAR-DEH]

Skadi is the hunter Goddess; the seeker and the finder. She has close associations with the Mountain Range and the Warrior Mystic. She is a third aspect to the Freya-Frigg relationship, being the shadow that is created by the light. Whenever we connect to either of the previous Goddess Essences, we see Skadi, for she is a necessary part of the process and creates an essential trinity within the Standing Stones context.

The amazing thing about this essence is that the perspective changes, depending on the situation, the point at which the essence is shifted to, and those involved. Like a shadow that changes in orientation and form, depending on the time of day, Skadi brings versatility to our treatments and practices.

Her influence is that in any treatment, practice or shifting to the essences of choice, there are unknown factors: things that cannot be known or have yet to be revealed. Usually these elements come into consciousness after the treatment or at some future point.

Turning our attention to the viewpoint of Skadi helps us identify where those shadows fall and provides a much greater level of definition to those shadows. This not only helps us provide a deeper level of pre-emptive treatment, but also helps us to work in situations where the root cause of dis-ease is elusive or hidden.

FRIGG [FRIK-KAR]

Frigg was the Queen of Asgard and her essence is of motherhood and birth. Similar in many ways to Freja, except Frigg's perspective is from a different layer of perception. She is of life, innocence, newness, and birth. Nonetheless, the selflessness and universal care that is offered by Freja is also that of Frigg.

As one shifts to the perspective of Frigg, there is often a heightened sense of prophecy and foresight, however, this can never be spoken of; it is secret knowledge that allows one to prepare, but not to change or redirect. For what we see from the vantage point of Frigg's gaze is what we must face to attain our goals, desires and life purpose. What we experience may be painful for us and for others, but with prior wisdom, we can create a journey that is smoother and eases the bruises we experience along the way.

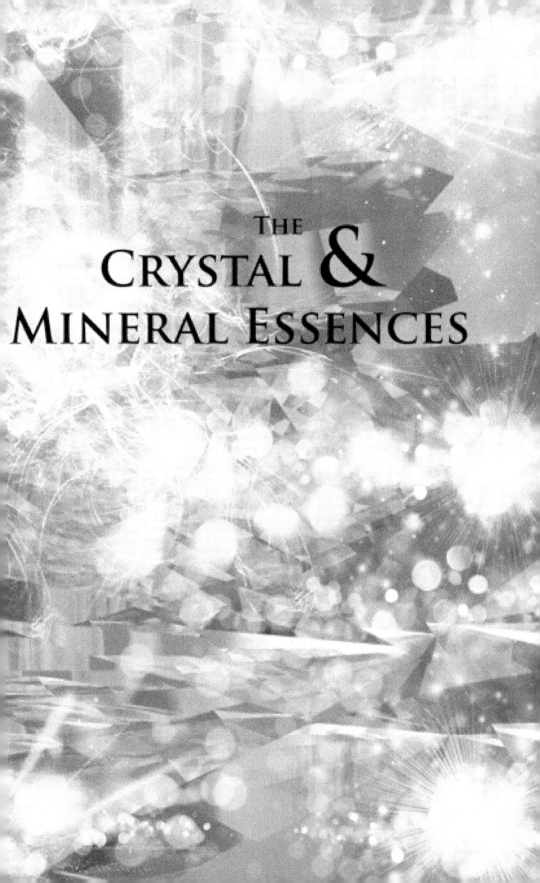

THE
CRYSTAL & MINERAL ESSENCES

Rose Quartz

Love is one of the major foundations of trauma, or rather, the lack of love – it is likely that you will know what it is to love somebody and yet, experience pain because of that love. You have probably experienced rejection, or loss, or grief, or the pain of unrequited love. Often, when a person is so lost in unrequited love or grief that they cannot see beyond it, adequate treatment is vital to help restore some form of equilibrium to that person's life.

Rose Quartz is one of the gentlest essences that help those who are fragile or emotionally delicate to a calm, almost disconnected state. Alleviating the pain they feel can cause them to seek out the source of this relief and create a strengthening of the connection between them and treatment. Once this has occurred you can continue to work with Rose Quartz or switch to another essence that will progress the treatment.

Amethyst

The Amethyst is well renowned for its healing and curative qualities, even as far back as the Ancient Greeks, who used the mineral as a defence against intoxication. Medieval soldiers used amethyst to protect them in battles and, in our technologically modern society, the mineral is valued in the electronics industry.

Amethyst not only helps one find peace and tranquillity of emotions and mind, it supports a strong attitude and can help ease depression. This essence can diminish anxiety and stops night terrors, whilst negating additions, especially that of alcohol. Physically, the Amethyst Essence is an excellent hangover cure, in addition to easing all forms of headache and pain. A universal healer, this essence can be worked with for a variety of dis-eases, from assisting with sleep disorders to improving skin condition and easing nausea.

Spiritually, the Amethyst Essence offers spiritual awakening, nurturing meditative practices, spiritual guidance and improves the healing qualities of other essences.

CITRINE

This golden-yellow mineral takes its name from the French 'Citron', meaning lemon. Used throughout history as a protective talisman, Citrine is said to 'transmute negative energy to positive' (a phrase that is inaccurate in Celtic Reiki terms) and this makes it popular today as a shield against disruptive emissions from electronic equipment. Much commercially available Citrine is actually Amethyst that has been artificially heated, as natural Citrine is much rarer.

Emotionally, the Citrine Essence eases depression, sadness, and releases negativity of thoughts and emotions. It transforms pessimism and works profoundly on the emotional layers of being. A calming, balancing essence, Citrine removes malice and vengeful thoughts, whilst offering space to reconcile the pains of the past.

Physically, the Essence of Citrine is fantastic at healing toxic shock and poisoning, as it is a powerful detoxifier. It also helps with: skin dis-ease; digestive issues; constipation; diabetes; and stomach problems, including ulcers. Spiritually, Citrine offers a more emotional spirituality (faith that is felt, rather than thought about) and changes contraction to expansion, whilst cleansing and clearing on all levels of being.

CLEAR QUARTZ

Quartz is a commonplace silicate that is anything but common in vibrancy and perspective. The powerful essence of Clear Quartz offers truly amazing healing potential, higher guidance, and an innate beauty in its simplicity.

This is the key to Clear Quartz; an uncomplicated focus on the treatment of physical issues, emotional trauma, cerebral challenge and spiritual conundrum. Whereas many essences have a very particular result or outcomes, the Clear Quartz is a generalist, yet it is quite astonishing how focused it is in its overall approach.

There is also a meeting of realms in the Clear Quartz Essence; the grounding of Earth and the refraction of light. Two vastly different layers of perception that meet in a single transitory glimpse of what we know (EarthLore) and what is unknown (EnergyLore).

This duality produces treatment benefits that are spiritually-orientated; conducted with a deep sense of wisdom and intuitive knowhow. Yet, treatments are also fully present in the physical world, solid in results and effects, as well as being long lasting. Thus, Clear Quartz is a favourite of Mystics and Masters alike; adaptable and flexible in usage, whilst always reliable. In other words, the Clear Quartz Essence is a universal treatment perspective that is centred on effect as opposed to cause, making it the essence of health, rather than an essence of particular dis-ease.

SMOKY QUARTZ

Similar in perspective to Clear Quartz, the Smoky Quartz Essence shifts focus slightly from universal healing to one of slight speciality. Here, there is an emphasis on the treatment of dis-ease and trauma where a person is particularly vulnerable or at risk in some way.

This could take the form of a trauma that was caused by an horrific event or action, which the person feels powerless to resolve or overcome. It could also be some issue that a person is embarrassed about or is ashamed of. (This might be totally 'assumed' on the part of the person or through the actual, callous reactions of others in the past). Whatever the individual details of the situation, Smoky Quartz will help a person to shift their awareness to self-empowerment and a realisation of personal responsibility.

This is multifaceted in value, for it internalises the cause and enables a person to do something about it—they may not have been to blame, but they can take responsibility to stop it from ever happening again, in addition to healing the effects, the foundation issue is having on them.

OBSIDIAN

The physical substance of Obsidian actually consists of the same material as Clear Quartz. The difference in appearance and texture, etc. comes from the way the two minerals are formed—one in the ground as part of natural rock formation, the other through the explosive actions of volcanoes. A volcanic glass, Obsidian is a beautiful contrast to Clear Quartz. They share much of the same perspective, yet there are differences.

The essence of Obsidian is much more nebulous than its clear cousin. Both perspectives deal with healing 'indiscriminately' though the Clear Quartz is simply a healer, without preference for the whys and wherefores; Obsidian works wonders for dis-ease and trauma that is actively hidden or evasive.

This could be viewed as a client not wanting to be healed, or actually relying on dis-ease in a sub-conscious way. It could also be that some journey of discovery is involved in the treatment, and therefore is actually an opportunity waiting to be found.

LABRADORITE

Labradorite is beautiful grey feldspar that displays amazing colours when held in the light: colours ranging from blues and green, to golden yellows and browns. The main features of Labradorite are its abilities to work with nightmares, night terror, and other sleep disorders. An excellent essence when used as a tonic to encourage peaceful, restful sleep. The essence relieves stress and anxiety, is brilliant at stopping panic attacks, and can be used in people who suffer from 'Night Nurses Paralysis'.

Spiritual transformation and deep insight are two keynote aspects of this essence that is quite unlike any other essence when working on expansion and spiritual growth. Just as this seemingly dull, grey rock lights up with beautiful colour when held in the light, its essence can bring the most amazing transformation, even when things seem drab and lacklustre.

JET

Whenever we experience the loss of somebody or something treasured, we go through a period of grieving in order to heal. Sometimes that process goes beyond healing and the emotion of grief itself becomes something to block out the loss.

When a person has been in sustained pain, the grief has a tendency to transcend love and may become a state in its own right. Here the person has felt the loss for so long, they actually forget the source of their emotion, favouring sorrow and pain as opposed to the original object of love/loss. It is in this situation that we turn to Jet.

Jet is a wonderful bearer of light and eases the pain of loss when it has stagnated and turned into bitterness, lack and resignation. It can also be used in cases of recent bereavement, easing shock and the different stages that follow. The amazing thing about this essence is that it enables the clearing and healing results of grief, whilst stabilising a person emotionally. Therefore, the grieving period becomes calmer and less trauma-instilling, whilst allowing a person to heal.

SAPPHIRE (BLUE AND PADPARADASHA)

Sapphires are stunning gems that exist in a range of colours from deep royal blue, to rich orange, powder blue, to vibrant lilac. The sapphire energy is cool and soothing, whilst also being invigorating for thoughts and creative processes, such as creative expression. The Sapphire Essence helps maintain a higher emotional function, softens violent, or overly-passionate emotions, and clears perceived blockages and obstacles.

On physiological levels, Sapphire reduces inflammation, lower fevers and heals burns. There is a connection between this essence and over-exposure to the sun, such as the ability of Sapphire to ease red, angry sunburn, alleviate heat stroke, and reduce dehydration – although this essence is no substitute for safety precautions when in the sun (such as drinking water and using a high-factor sun cream!).

Sapphire develops spiritual creativity and brings out intuitive abilities, and is an essential meditation aid for those who enjoy synaesthesia and lots of visuals.

EMERALD

The rich green mineral is a form of beryl that is highly prized as a precious gem, second only to diamond. As a therapeutic essence, Emerald also has many beneficial properties that make it an essential addition for every practitioner.

These include: a great calming effect on the nervous system, disconnection from feelings of revenge; assisting those who have experienced trauma, especially regarding to one's parents; those who behave in an arrogant and egotistical manner; and people who are prone to react in error to what is said.

There are many physiological aspects to the Emerald perspective also, for it eases the effects of mental illness, including Down's syndrome and Alzheimer's disease. It is a valuable essence in the treatment of those who have suffered strokes and for the effects of cancer treatments, such as radiation treatments. Emerald's perspective is reported to focus on the circulatory, lymph, and digestive systems, in addition to the kidneys, liver and heart. An eclectic essence, Emerald helps issues from itchy skin to epilepsy and eyesight distortions.

Spiritually, Emerald Essence helps people who have experienced a loss of faith, those who feel lost and bewildered and individuals who want to heal the world, but have not recognised their need to heal themselves.

MORGANITE

Morganite is a beautiful pink form of beryl that is mined in Brazil. The delicate pink colour is created by the inclusion of manganese in the formation process and it is this sumptuous hue that makes Morganite so sought after. The qualities of Morganite are usually 'heart and chest centred', both physically and emotionally, as the essence enhances compassion and empathy, nurtures self-control, and eases the pain of separation from a loved one. Morganite Essence is an emotional balancer that inspires patience for those in a rush and motivates those who feel stuck. The essence has been noted to help heal Emphysema, Tuberculosis, heart disease, and breathing problems, including Asthma.

This essence has many spiritual qualities as well, including increased spiritual insight and wisdom, connection to higher intelligence and ancient ancestral wisdom that is locked away in deep-layers of the psyche.

Aquamarine

This beautiful light blue/green mineral was once imbued with the energy of the ocean and often treasured by sailors, who believed it would bestow them with bravery and safe passage through the mightiest of storms. A form of beryl, these stones are often valued more in modern times as jewellery.

On emotional and cerebral layers, the Aquamarine Essence soothes the mind, calms fears and phobias, aids recovery from depression, boosts confidence, increases self-awareness and stimulates courage and strength. This essence is also fantastic at alleviating a fear of drowning and with the Essence, Blue, removes seasickness and general nausea.

Physically, this essence works on all throat issues, laryngitis, loss of voice, etc. and is very helpful to singers and those who use their voice a lot. It is additionally conducive for the lymph system and strengthens the Immune System. Aquamarine centres and balances spiritual awareness, particularly in connection to the ocean and Furthest Ocean (realm). It helps us to find direction on all layers and is particularly helpful in relation to sea travel.

IRON

The essence of Iron creates boundaries and thus enables disconnection from habitual perspectives. Of course, these boundaries are merely an illusion of viewpoint, created from taking the forceful, dense characteristics of Iron as a physical substance and defining the same qualities 'energetically'.

Used for centuries as an 'etheric disruptor' (disrupting of energetic vibrations), iron and its essence create chaos, without any other result. Thus, the Iron Essence will be followed by other essences (unless the purpose of the treatment/practice is chaos!) that restore some form of harmony or order. Usually, Silver Essence is preferred when treating habitual behaviour, however, when Silver is producing the wanted feedback, Iron forms a deeper perspective and action.

This essence is an excellent repatterning agent that will frequently wipe away unwanted sensations, clearing residual perspectives and eliminating unwanted environmental associations, (where a person or people associate contractive responses with an environment or place – this might often be described as a haunting or unwanted 'presence').

COPPER

Copper is symbolic of vibrant energy and mental agility. This beautiful red-orange metal is very distinctive and highly prized in the electronic/technology industries for its electrical conductive ability. Copper is often worn as a bracelet to purify the blood and help with the relief of arthritis and is an essential mineral for life. All these qualities are mirrored in the perspective of the Copper Essence, which brings mental agility, quick wit, improved memory and increased speed of reaction, as well as acting as a physical healing agent in cases of arthritis, rheumatism, lethargy and tiredness. Copper Essence also cleanses the blood and is an excellent pain reliever, especially with broken bones.

GOLD

This soft, yellow metal has long been revered and much sought after for its beauty and rarity. This is reflected in the Gold Essence, which is derived from the harvest of rare Welsh Gold, which came from the same mine as that of the Crown jewels.

Regarded as a universal healer, gold has also been coveted for its ability to heal 'all ails'. The essence encompasses an overall healing ability, for example: assisting people to gain a meaningful value for wealth and richness; eases materialism, or an over-acquisitive nature; stops gambling addiction; enhances prosperity, true abundance, and a healthy attitude towards money; enables the expression of higher mental and emotional processes; as an anti-depressant and general therapeutic tonic/healer.

SILVER

There are two chaotic essences in the Standing Stones, Iron and Silver. Whilst Iron thrives purely on chaos, Silver is an essence that results in harmony and order through chaos. Both Iron and Silver work by 'shaking-up' fixed or locked patterns, habits, addictions, themes, etc.

When some action or connection has been repeated many times and has become fixed, trying to shift the situation may result in temporary change, before reverting back, or no change at all. Silver (and Iron) disrupt all patterns in a defined area, enabling drastic change to occur. Once in chaos and 'flux', the Silver Essence will bring harmony and stabilisation to the situation, offering a base to further treatment and definition.

Steeped in tradition and an integral part of folklore, Silver is also of great use when working with those who are dogmatic or victims of religious dogma. People who are experiencing long-term difficulties through what they have been told in the past, or the past action of others, often need to lose their way in order to find it again. Silver offers both parts of the journey.

OPAL

Opal is often perceived as an unlucky stone, for contrasting reasons, although many of these do trace back to conjecture and personal opinion. One particular thought is that if Opals are not regularly brought into contact with water they dry up, contract and fall from jewellery, thus being lost. It is said that only those born under the star sign of Libra may wear the stone, as Opal is their birthstone. It is therefore interesting to note that Opal essence has many properties that suggest 'luck-inducing' qualities, with reports of an increased rate of goal manifestation and general 'lucky' events.

The Opal Essence enhances memory, brings emotional wellbeing, releases inhibitions and is reported to bring pleasant dreams. There are also elements of inspiration and imagination enhancement in this perspective. Physically the essence has a high feedback of helping dis-ease of the nervous system, such as Parkinson's, Motor Neurone, etc. It can improve eyesight and help ease dis-eases of the eyes.

IOLITE

The Iolite Essence works mainly on higher cerebral and spiritual levels, displaying remarkable qualities when enhancing meditation and inner-vision, synaesthesia, etc. This dark blue/purple mineral is renowned for its polarising qualities, appearing colourless at certain angles. Iolite works wonders on psychological addictions, where a person has a compulsive need of a substance, action, and so on, but the source of the addiction is not actually physically addictive. It is also a good essence to use when wishing to do vision work, or dreamtime.

Physically, the essence is a great hangover cure and greatly decreases the effects of alcohol. Iolite also heals the sinuses, throat dis-eases and skin disorders, such as blistering and warts. Spiritually, there is a lot of feedback to support the psychic enhancement produced by this essence, which also strengthens meditation and spiritual vision.

GARNET

This enchanting semi-precious gem can be found in colours ranging from a rich wine-red, to vibrant brown, and even fiery orange. Coveted for its grounding and protective qualities, Garnet is also a wonderfully healing stone that focuses on the heart, lungs and blood. It increases passionate energy, supporting emotional intensity and is excellent for people who are cut off emotionally. Useful as a blood cleanser, Garnet heals the vascular system and can ease respiratory dis-ease, according to common feedback.

PLUTONIUM

Plutonium is fast acting and very efficient at creating the perceived, total disconnection from any physical environment, dynamic or situation. Rather than simply changing perspective, this essence causes a state that is not viable in 'entropy' where the two perspectives (person and dynamic) cannot connect, because of some Universal impossibility.

An important aspect of entropy is where certain actions become impossible, for example, imagine you could travel back in time; it would be impossible for you to cause any action that would stop you from being born, because you would then not exist to go back and cause that action! The Plutonium Essence alters perspective to viewpoints where entropy means that a complete disconnection takes place—it is impossible for you to be connected to that dynamic, situation, etc.

In traditional terminology this might have been known as 'protection', however there is a major difference between defending or protecting against some detrimental influence and actually making it a Universal impossibility for you to encounter that influence.

Salt

Used in physical ways to cleanse and heal, salt also provides us with a superb purifier from an energetic perspective, acting particularly well in the realms of suppressed feelings and thoughts. Salt has a relatively brusque or harsh action in the way it works, because it practically forces the emotions that need attention to the surface.

Some people experience a huge amount of suppression in life, not only in the dominion of emotions, but also with religious denomination, spirituality, love, sexual orientation, health, dis-ease, and many other areas that others may deem to be culturally or socially unacceptable. The need to hide one's true nature at all cost can produce those who hide or feel inadequate. They lurk out of sight, forgotten in the shadows, wanting to so much be accepted but remain unable to find that acceptance.

A salt perspective will heal people on these levels, so that other, more soothing essences can then be applied in the usual way. The Salt Essence can also be used to alter the perspective of locations or areas that seem disruptive in some way, or the destructive dynamics that form between people.

Arsenic

This dull, grey metal is highly poisonous in physical form, though in contrast, its essence is deeply healing for heart dis-ease, issues with the blood and circulation, and the respiratory system. The Arsenic Essence has an integrally spiritual effect, creating radical detoxification on a physical level to help enlightenment and spiritual growth.

The essence works wonders when combined with the poisons from the Woodland Realm or when used with other Crystal Essences of the Standing Stones.

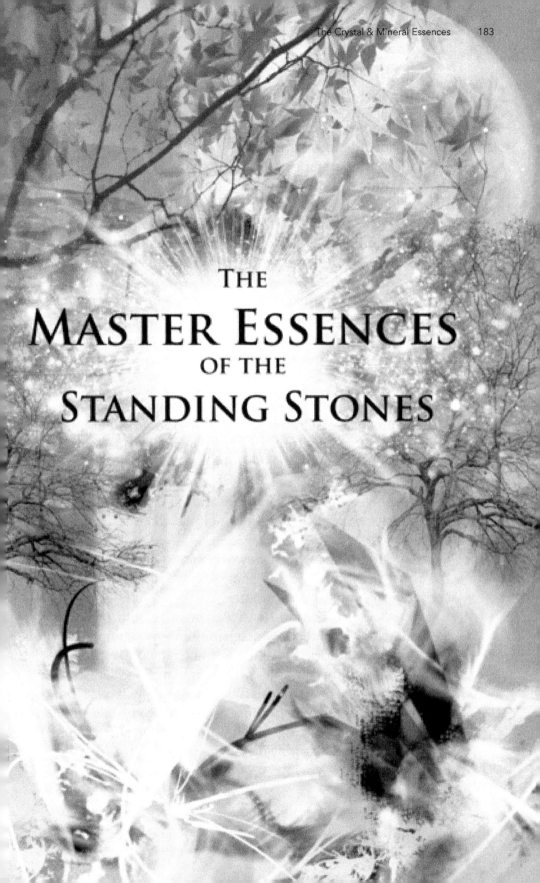

THE
MASTER ESSENCES
OF THE
STANDING STONES

Aesc – AE—Odin—(AE-S)

The essence of the visionary and leader; this is the Master Nordic and Runic Essence. The perspective of the Norse God Odin, this perspective is shifted to when conducting the Orientation to the Standing Stones and the essences of this realm.

Encapsulated in this essence is the viewpoint of truth, wisdom and the power to inspire others—this is the perspective of the one who changes the world, creates a legacy, and does what few have done before. There is a core of powerful communication and the ability to convey important messages; the master orator. There is enthusiasm, charisma and a nature charm that heals and inspires on mere contact.

Lemurian Seed Crystal

The Lemurian Seed Crystal is a very rare form of clear quartz that has a slight pink tint, caused by minute quantities of iron that were captured during the crystal's formation. The crystal is believed to be 'seeded' with information from the ancient Lemurian civilization and could be viewed as a 'gateway' or device that connects us to other layers of intelligence.

The essence of this awe-inspiring crystal is one of the most powerful and life-changing of all essences. It is certainly the most transformative of the Crystal Essences. The therapies of Lemuria and Atlantis4D (both now part of Celtic Reiki practice), Ascension Energy Therapy and the Viridian Method, are all based, in part, on knowledge gleaned during meditations with Lemurian Seed Crystals.

With such a truly astounding legacy, it was only natural that the essence of these remarkable crystals would become the Master Essence for the Crystal and Mineral Essences, as well as playing a vital role in the Standing Stones Realm.

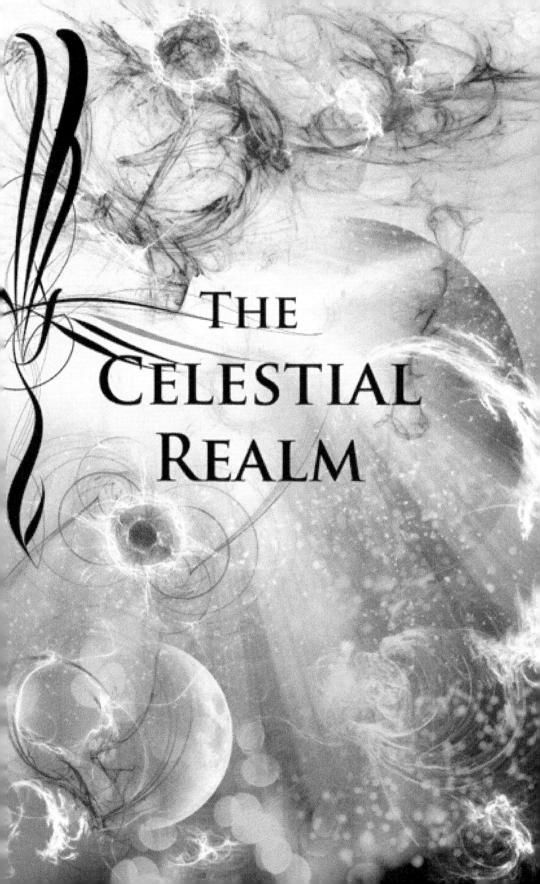

The
Celestial
Realm

THE
STELLAR
ESSENCES

ARIES

The essence of Aries is that of independence, forward-thinking, motivation and energy. With the perspective of constant motion, this essence is always pushing towards some result or goal; it does so with potency and sheer magnetism.

An excellent choice when treating stagnation, lethargy, or lack of motivation, Aries can also be used to treat aggression and destructive anger. In these instances, the essence does not remove the anger, but re-focuses it into positive action and transmutes aggression into assertion.

There is a real indication that the Aries Essences has the greatest influence on emotional and cerebral levels; helping people to overcome challenging times and offering strength of conviction when a person does not really know their own mind. This is the perspective of passion, not only in a physical sense, but in the behaviour of being passionate about a cause or activity.

Spiritually, and upon the conscious layers of the psyche, Aries can help people to overcome inertia at the beginning of some new venture, or after periods of rest and inactivity. Gathering force quickly and powerfully, a person will not only experience motivation, willpower and renewed courage, they will be propelled through limitations and obstacles quickly and painlessly.

The Aries Essence has many connections both within the Celestial Realm and from the other Celtic Reiki Realms. These include: the Mars Essence; the Elemental Essence, Fire; the Colour Essence of Red; Fearn and Garnet, to name but a few.

The essence is also cardinal, meaning it is both progressive and expansive, as well as having the greatest influence on the 'self' when issues are personally focused.

TAURUS

The Taurean perspective is of physical strength, determination and stamina. If Aries gets things done from the viewpoint of energetic motivation and Leo through enthusiasm, the Taurus Essence does what it does through the force of will alone, or what some might call 'bloody-mindedness'! It brings a sense of rigidity to the essence that works wonders with people who find it challenging to stick to one path or goal, or those whose behaviour is fickle and capricious.

This essence instils a sense of stability for those who find it challenging to trust others and will be a bedrock for those battered by the storm. Yet the Taurus Essence is also beautiful in aesthetic and deed. An inspiration to artists, emotional depth for singers and an all-enveloping compassion for healers, the essence has connection to Venus, the essence of beauty.

Another aspect of the Taurus Essence is that of foresight and taking the time to think things through. Of course, there are occasions in life when we simply need to 'take the plunge', however if a client (or oneself) favours rash behaviour, without adequate deliberation, Taurus can help a person stand back from their current situation and take a moment to think through their actions. This is particularly useful for those who speak before they think and end up offending others or losing out on something that a period of reflection might have attained for them.

The essence of Taurus has connections to the Elemental Essence of Earth, The Oceanic Essence of Pink and Saille. As a 'fixed' perspective, it leans towards the physical world and is a wonderful manifestation essence that is very focused on material possessions. Conversely, Taurus is also very connected to the essences of beauty, love and loyalty, such as: Quert, Onn, Plane, Arbutus, Green and Clear Quartz.

GEMINI

The essence of Gemini is communicative and intellectual, with an integral theme of duality. This lends the essence to those who need to see the world beyond themselves or to understand another's point of view. This is not necessarily 'empathy', but logical comprehension of a different perspective. If the essence of Taurus facilitates a steady path and fixed goals, Gemini is the opposite; creating a meandering of focus and the ability to be aware of many different choices, results and methods.

The connections of this essence span the planetary (Mercury), the elemental (Air), and the Oceanic (Yellow), as well as having close ties to Huathe. As a mutable essence, the dynamics of its perspective are ever-changing and multifaceted. It is the dancer around the Maypole and the dabbled glinting of sunlight within a gemstone.

The Gemini Essence can help one to know one's own limitations and move beyond them through the creation of new ideas and concepts. The Gemini perspective gets results through innovation, adaptation and lateral thinking. It can also help those who need clarity when many contrasting and even conflicting factors are at play. This is especially useful in situations where there are two challenges that are polar opposites. The light and the dark, the eternal and the fleeting, the minute and the huge; all become integrated with the use of Gemini.

Using this essence when in social or formal situations can enhance the ability to think on one's feet, become an excellent orator and inspire with new and innovative insights into old challenges. It improves the ability to convey complex ideas and assists when treating people who have issues with communicating on a one-to-one basis or when confronted by a large group of people.

CANCER

This intuitive, emotional and highly empathic perspective is essential when treating those who want to become more in-tune with their feelings. Mysterious and hidden, the Cancerian viewpoint is connected to Water and the Moon/Thea, as well as sharing many similar traits to Green and Duir. Yet, we can also see touches of the Cancer Essence in Llochw, Obsidian, and Mor.

The ability of this essence to melt barriers and boundaries, to penetrate the most hardened of hearts and minds is phenomenal. For, if Gemini is cerebral and Taurus physical, the essence of Cancer is heartfelt emotion. This manifests in a romanticised or wistful way, as opposed to passion; the fairytale and nostalgic are of far greater importance in the action of this essence than the more base emotions.

Cancer is one of the best essences to shift to when treating families, broken relationships or those who feel unloved and alone. There is such a sense of care and compassion with this essence that immersion within its soft folds is rather like being held and gently rocked, whilst listening to the soothing words of a lullaby.

A cardinal essence, Cancer is expansive and seeks to achieve some form of 'betterment'; whether this be more love or kindness, a greater sense of security and stability, or the nurture of home. For home is sacred in the Cancer perspective and there is no essence better at treating one's home or living environment. Cancer brings a sense of comfort and harmony to the home and helps us settle into a new home or enhance our sense of belonging in our existing home.

Another valuable aspect of the Cancer Essence is its intuitive qualities that help when combined with other perspectives to increase the level of insight in a treatment or manifestation scenario. This not only offers foresight and prophecy, but a sense of assurance and inner-knowing.

LEO

The application of the Leo Essence in treatment is magnetic and will cause good things to gravitate towards the those involved in the treatment. As they shift to the Leo perspective, they are often overwhelmed by the cheerful and enthusiastic wave of energy that washes over them. This is the essence of Leo; a passionate, charismatic perspective that enchants those who connect to it.

There is a sense of authority in the essence that makes it excellent for those in a position of leadership, especially people who need to lead others, even when reluctant to do so, or doubtful of their own abilities. Creating a natural charm that makes one's presence strangely magnetic to others, Leo provides those who would normally go unnoticed with an indescribable and intangible 'something'. It is this quality that we follow in others and feel pride about in ourselves.

As well as bringing a certain performance to a person's natural presence, Leo presents us with gravitas and focuses us on the strength of our convictions. Principled and forthright, we become stronger in mind, spirit, and passion when we walk from the Leo viewpoint.

Leo has affinities with the Sun, Fire, and the essence of Gold. The Leo perspective is close to Orange and its assertive role as a guardian, places the essence close to Tinne. A fixed essence, Leo is strong and secure; unshakable, even in the face of adversity.   W h e n working with the perspective of Leo, you can be creative with the dynamic it creates in treatment, manifestation, etc. The essence of Leo literally magnetises and pulls things to a central point—the focus of treatment. So if you are manifesting, the essence will pull in situations, tools, people, and so on that help to create a desired outcome. In healing treatments, the essence will also entice the needed environmental, substance, and energetic requirements to heal dis-ease. When you keep the method of Leo in mind, you can adapt it to whatever your particular needs are in any situation.

VIRGO

The Virgo Essence is fixed in the idea of perfection and when working from its perspective, there is a definite focus on creating the ideal in any situation. The essence is not only cleansing and detoxifying (to clear away the unwanted), it also prepares and creates the way for perfection to arrive. When considering the viewpoint of Virgo, words such as 'truth', 'precision' and 'elegance' come to mind. There is an additional air of excellence when dealing with the Virgo perspective, which is continually pushing the focus of the treatment to strive beyond its current range. This makes it an exceptional choice when treating high-achiever who wish to better themselves, however, perhaps this essence is best avoided when treating those who are not coping with (or meeting) the expectations they have set themselves.

This essence was truly made to help those who want to be of service to others. Where a person's aim is to please or support other people (perhaps even more than the self), a shifting of perspective to that of Virgo will facilitate the best (most effective and efficient) means of doing this.

The discovery (or rediscovery) of purity is a common effect of this essence, where the focus of treatment will often report a simplicity or deep sense of being pure as the essence integrates with them. This can result in a person becoming critical of others or noticing 'mistakes' to a greater degree, yet when a person is truly in-tune with the essence, they relax and enjoy the almost utopian embrace of this beautiful vista.

The connections this essence has with essences from the other Celtic Reiki Realms include: the Earth element, Coll, Muin, Red and Green in combination and Mercury. As a mutable essence there needs to be a degree of flexibility when working with Virgo, as a rigid approach may result in a treatment or action that is too reliant on a particular result to notice the other successes that have been attained.

LIBRA

This is the essence of beauty, purity and harmony. The Libra Essence is firmly fixed from the viewpoint of justice and natural lore; wanting to create fairness and harmony for all. Yet the unusual thing about the essence is that its cardinal nature means that this static, everlasting and absolutely fixed point, is always pushing outwards and expanding. This result can leave others flummoxed by its behaviour, yet a simple way of understanding how this can be is that Libra is transitory in an expansive way—it is fixed in the moment and each moment is more than before.

Work with the essence of Libra today and you will find an absolute truth, work with it again tomorrow and that same truth will be more evolved and sometimes very different in appearance. This does not invalidate the essence's nature, it simply confines it to the immediate period of time and space.

The essence of Libra is excellent when working with legal situations. relationship issues and matters of the heart. It also creates a keen eye for the aesthetically pleasing and the sensual. For those who want to be more romantic, charming, or refined, the Libran Essence will offer these in abundance!

The dynamics of the Libran perspective create close affinity with the element of Air, the essences of blue and Gort. It also shares much with Opal, Venus and any essence that deals with balance, harmony and relationships.

The Libra viewpoint will help a person to see both sides of an argument, act as peacemaker or bring a more harmonious feel to any situation. For those who are stuck in dogma or rigid thinking, this essence brings a gust of wind to blow away the cobwebs and helps them to change their opinions to ease the workings of social, relationship and even business interactions. The true diplomat of the essences, eloquence, charm and a certain mystery are all an integral part of the Libra Essence that can be tapped into if required.

SCORPIO

Scorpio is intensely emotional and completely encompasses the entire emotional spectrum; from rapture to despair, love to hatred, the ethereal to the base. This mirrors the polarity of the Scorpio viewpoint, from the darkest of depths to the highest states of exhilaration. Therefore, the essence is excellent at treating extremes and lack of extreme alike. The essence will counteract any extreme mood or behaviour by shifting to the polar opposite and it will take any instance of nonchalance of lack of feeling and inspire to new heights. This makes it excellent at treating depression, grief, lethargy, or emotional numbness.

The Scorpio Essence is similar in viewpoint to the Dwr Essence, Magenta and Red Essences, Ngetal and Ruby. Its fixed outlook is paired with Pluto and focused upon the mysteries of life, death and beyond.

The Scorpio Essence is secretive and shares the Keeper of Secrets status with Fearn; this denotes wonderful results when working with hidden dis-ease or situations where a doctors have been unable to offer a diagnosis based on symptoms. Powerful and transformative, the essence of Scorpio is of sex, birth, life, and death. It also encapsulates the mysteries that surround each and can be used to help a person unravel their own, private puzzles.

When you shift to the perspective of Scorpio, be prepared to sense the power, emotion and 'edginess' of the view. It can be all-consuming, heart-pounding, joyous, ascending and potent in sensation, yet there is a very palpable knowledge that this could take us in either direction. Poles are poles, they are neither good, nor bad, just different. Most people, however, have a conscious preference for one or the other, so be aware of which pole you are moving towards when using this essence.

SAGITTARIUS

If ever an essence personified the ability of people to reach for their dreams and make them reality, it is that of Sagittarius. This really is one perspective that invites you to reach for the stars and bring them back to Earth in a blaze of fiery light. Ever on the quest of originality and something new, this essence brings a freshness and originality to our outlook. This essence is of the free spirit, the adventurer, the hunter and the seeker; it provides us with the desire to see new horizons and distant shores.

Sagittarius is similar in outlook to Jupiter, the Tan Essence, Violet and Ruis. Its mutable nature brings the spirit of adventure and a need for new, contrasting experiences. Philosophy, religion and learning are all of deep importance in this perspective, making the essence an enhancer of intelligence and knowledge.

The perspective of the Sagittarius Essence comes with a real optimism that is contagious. Rather like a party that goes with a bang, where people simply click and the atmosphere is electric, this essence provides an electricity that motivates people into action—the action of getting what they want, achieving more, and creating excellence in their life. When working from the viewpoint of Sagittarius, it is rather like having a little voice on your shoulder, whispering words of encouragement and positive affirmation in your ear. The difference being that the little voice is like thunder and the affirmations arrive with the force of a hurricane!

This essence is also excellent for people who tend not to give very much. Receiving is like the flow of the stream; if you block the path of the stream, the flow is decreased along the entire length of the stream. By nurturing the generosity and desire to give within a person, this essence increases the flow of receiving for all.

CAPRICORN

Beith is the essence that bears many of the Capricorn themes, although this may not be immediately obvious. The Capricorn Essence is about long-term benefits as opposed to immediate results. This essence will help a person to set out on an on-going adventure, always focusing on little steps to great dreams.

With the essence of Beith, new beginnings are highlighted and it is the integrity and potential of these beginnings where we find the common ground in the two perspectives. If a blueprint is designed with the future in mind, it will have a clear focus on the steps ahead which sustain a journey, rather than a quick sprint to success.

Beith also set us on our new adventurers with adequate 'supplies' for the road ahead. If we understand Beith as birth and new life, we would want that life (and that newness) to be with us as long as possible, so Beith is not simply encompassment of those first few weeks and months, it sets us up with everything we need until the end of a task or life. Capricorn's emphasis is on the regulated use of the things we need.

Tradition, convention and the tried and trusted path are all of value in the Capricorn perspective. Initiation is also an integral part of this viewpoint, for as we embark on any new venture, the wisdom of old and the ability to instil any plan with the utmost chance of success deserves some ritual or respectful action to state that 'this is a worthwhile journey'.

The Capricorn perspective shares much with the Saturn Essence, Indigo, Pridd and Obsidian, for each of these essences share the qualities of higher vision, longevity, perseverance, and guardianship through all the perceived challenges and 'perils' of life. There is a pessimistic streak that is engrained into the Capricorn essence, and whilst this may be of lacklustre to the optimist, when treating those who are often disappointed in life, love and success, this can help the art of preparation and planning for any eventuality.

AQUARIUS

The idealistic essence of Aquarius is associated with communities; focusing on groups that range in size from the small family to the largest cultural, political and social societies. Yet, this is not a traditional approach to the way of things, for Aquarius is non-conformist and offbeat in perspective. This essence brings with it a progressive viewpoint that challenges convention, revolutionises beliefs and changes the world.

Associated with the essence of Uranus, White, Amethyst and Luis, the Aquarian Essence's fixed approach to life offers a paradox that is shared by the three Stellar Essences that have an Annal influence. The Aquarius viewpoint is fixated on being completely unexpected and is static in only one aspect: its ability to never be where you think it is! This seemingly whimsical, almost flaky appearance of the essence could make it the butt of all jokes, however there is an intrinsic value in the Aquarius perspective.

Aquarius Essence brings idealism and visionary potential. It enables the narrow-minded to expand their vision and those at a loss for ideas to revolutionise their way of perceiving the world. Creative in an innovative manner and unique in every nuance, the essence brings independence to the weak and co-dependent, lateral thinking to those stuck in a groove and emancipation to those who have been deprived from freedom of thought, will, or action.

The viewpoint of invention, this essence complements essences that can be used at the beginning of a process or venture; it can also quieten fears and trepidation through the shifting of perspective and philosophies. The perspective of Aquarius will enable the focus of any treatment to see things in a completely unconventional way; to notice what others have missed; and to structure their internal representation of the world unlike other people.

PISCES

The intangible fleeting and flitting of fishes personifies the nature of the Piscean perspective. Akin to Dwr, Cyan, Amethyst and the Planetary Essence of Neptune, there are many aquatic themes at the core of this essence. A mutable perspective, Pisces is both mystical and intuitive sharing many qualities with Nuin. Any 'entity' that exists in the physical world, comes about through definition and more precisely, two types of definition; the 'internal' definition and the 'external' definition. These act as an inner will, which pushes against the world and an external force that resists the push. These two dynamics offer balance and stability. Pisces is both of these forces, constantly pushing and pulling, compelling and resisting.

This perspective provides the ability to be happy in one's own skin, to step away from the world and reflect in solitude, or to be in the midst of great crowds, the life and soul of any party and very much the supporter of others in times of need. In this respect, the essence shares much with the other dual essences of Libra and Gemini.

Through the polarity of the Pisces Essence comes another paradox, inasmuch as it forms an inability to distinguish the separateness of the world from oneself. The Piscean approach is one that understands internal thoughts to be the absolute truth and indicative of all things in the world. Thus it makes an excellent essence for treatment in those who feel isolated or different in some way. It also is an essential part of progression into the social spheres of higher expansion, such as the Experiential Sphere and beyond.

The Pisces Essence is also a perfect choice for those who tend to set their sight lower than their capacity; rather than propelling themselves to greater layers of achievement and excellence, they 'make do' and 'put up' with what they believe their 'lot in life' presents them with.

THE
PLANETARY
ESSENCES

MERCURY

The essence of Mercury is highly cerebral in nature and focused upon communication and education. Once you have shifted to the Mercury perspective, there is a sense of authority and of being in a position of knowledge. This is not associated with government or 'dominance', but a sense of being the source of guidance and wisdom for others. This sensation is what a teacher feels when standing to address their class, or how a wise Master experiences the act of speaking their truth to students.

There is an innate and complex logic to the Mercury perspective, which is rather like an energetic form of the personal development therapies based upon communication and thought (NLP, Coaching, etc.). Patterns and methodologies are highlighted which enables this essence to work well with compulsive or habitual behaviour, to break repetitive cycles that are damaging to health and instil new behavioural patterns which support a person's overall wellbeing.

The Mercury Essence can improve the flow of thought and is a wonderfully nurturing essence for authors, journalists, editors and anybody who works with words. The essence also has close links to other highly intellectual, thought-based professions and as such, can be of immense assistance when working with doctors, judges, philosophers, mathematicians, scientists and a whole manner of other professionals that may find the ideas behind the Mercury Essence more challenging than the dis-ease or emotional issue they are facing! Mercury will therefore ease their passage into treatment and create a buffer that softens the transition from left hand brain to right.

This perspective is the initiator of journeys and after using the essence of Mercury, you may find that some form of travel is necessary for the treatment or practice to take full effect. This could be a trip to discover something that will help you or a relaxing holiday, either way, the travel will be unusual in some way and very thought provoking!

VENUS

The nature of Venus is that of love and beauty. The essence has a profound effect in any practice or treatment that involves relationships, sex, business partnerships, and creativity. The perspective of aesthetes, Venus not only harmonises the way that people integrate with and get along with each other, it also brings out the beauty in any situation. When applied to a situation or particular challenge, the Venus Essence not only works to balance out contractive dynamics and form a harmonising influence, it will also make the results look, feel and seem more beautiful and sensual.

This abundant trait of the Venus Essence makes it an excellent choice of perspective at the end of a treatment or practice. After other essences have been aligned with to conduct highly specialised treatments and finely-honed results, the Venus Essence can then conclude the treatment, tying any 'loose-ends' and smoothing over rough edges, until all is looking beautiful.

In its own right, Venus is the perfect choice for supporting and healing relationships between people, be they intimate, social or business. Yet there is another valuable reason to work with this essence in treatment and that is to heal the relationship one has with oneself. Venus is a self-treatment essence that integrates the self, and hence, could be seen as the essence of choice when wanting to discover self-love and for seeing the beauty within oneself.

The Essence of artists, healers, designers, beauticians, and anybody whose profession is centred on making things of beauty or increasing love and compassion in the world. Yet, the layers of Venus that create wealth and abundance also make it a great essence for entrepreneurs and people who wish to turn their passion or joy into their main source of income. Venus is like gold dust in these instances, bringing success and prosperity to those who choose to spend their time doing what they are in love with.

MARS

The essence of Mars is very physical in nature and shares many of the same qualities as Orange. The sexuality and physical activity of the essence mean that it is one of the most effective to work from when you are treating any issue of a sexual nature, physical injury or when increasing fitness levels.

Mars is excellent at inspiring to action, invigorating and stirring deep seated emotions that compel us to achieve some goal or ideal. For people who have given up or feel the road ahead is simply too challenging, Mars renews strength, taps into inner reserves of courage and gives the force of might to those who are downtrodden.

This perspective is forceful and powerful; there is no meandering here, simply focus and direct action. This makes it beneficial for those who need to be assertive, to say "no" or to stick to their principles. The essence will also improve overall confidence and self-assurance, enabling one to take decisive action and to discern the right choices in any given situation. The ability to think on one's feet in this way is essential for those in positions of leadership and mastery.

One noteworthy effect of the Mars Essence is that it is incredibly hot and will warm those who use it, rather like a hot flush! This means that it is a remarkable analgesic, with excellent pain relief properties. These include: headache, back pain, muscular and joint injuries, strains and sprains, etc.

The viewpoint of Mars will offer discipline to those who have difficulty in finishing things and stamina to people who feel they cannot go on to complete a task or personal mission. It provides energy to those who are lethargic or exhausted. All in all, Mars improves health, increases vitality, heightens energy and enables us to get things done.

JUPITER

Jupiter's perspective is of growth and expansion, which creates the dynamic of increasing, evolving, and developing everything that is shifted to the Jupiter view. Increasing prosperity, wealth and 'riches' in a universal sense, rather than simple monetary terms, this essence is excellent for anybody who is dissatisfied with their current circumstances.

The Jupiter Essence also nurtures expanded layers of perception and thought, from higher education and learning, to spirituality and higher wisdom. Encompassing areas such as morality and a personal sense of right and wrong, Jupiter helps us to do what is best for all, instead of doing what we are told.

Jupiter is exploration of the unknown and discovery of invaluable wisdom; it is life-changing and awe-inspiring. For, wherever there is some word or action that transforms, there is the essence of Jupiter.

In addition there is a wonderful duality about the Jupiter Essence, because, whilst Jupiter has a gravitas that seems serious in tone and nature, it also encourages a sense of fun, merry-making and joviality. Child-like in so many ways, the view of Jupiter is one of curiosity and wonder; everything being looked at, touched, listened to, and explored with an insatiable hunger for understanding. This passion is not necessarily an intellectual one, although it does centre on the mind, it is more a passionate adventure, a game played by a child that offers exuberant fun, but also teaches valuable lessons in the playing.

Celtic Reiki Masters may find Jupiter particularly useful when teaching, as this dual process of higher learning and the rapture of play are a very special part of the Celtic Reiki learning process for students and teachers alike!

SATURN

The perspective of Saturn could be viewed as the polar opposite of Jupiter, for this is the viewpoint of contraction and limitation. Yet, this is not in itself a contractive dynamic, for Saturn offers us the ability to scale-down when needed and to define anew. We all face times when we take on too much, acquire too much, experience too much; times when we just want to let go and be for a while. Saturn is the essence than can help us do this: to contract inwards to our core-self and redefine who we are and our purpose in life.

Another wonderful aspect of Saturn is its ability to help us create the intangible in the physical world. Whenever we imagine or dream about our desires, they exist in some greatly expanded state, beyond the physical world—they exist, but we cannot sense them with our five solid-based senses. Saturn works with the act of definition to help us put parameters on our goals and wants, so that we make them physical.

Saturn's perspective is practical, logical and what some might call 'realistic'. Despite this, Saturn is a real example of everything in its place. For this essence is not the dreamer, not the creator, not the inspiration, or the source—it is the worker that produces, the craftsman that makes, the mechanic that assembles and the accountant that balances the books.

This translates to a valuable opportunity for those who are creative or imaginative, yet cannot seem to bring their ideas into fruition. The artist that never finishes a painting, the author who never finds the time to write, the entrepreneur who cannot find the money to start a business, or visionary who is unable to find people to listen... Saturn brings practical, physical answers to where there was only ever thought or visualisation.

URANUS

This perspective is unusual and unconventional in essence; it facilitates a perception of all things that not only goes against the traditional or commonly-accepted ways, it starts from a different place altogether! Hence, the Uranus Essence is inventive, provocative and revolutionary. For those who are stuck through their own limitations or the rules prescribed to them through society, Uranus will strip away barriers and create a completely alternative method of thought.

Everybody has specific personality traits that mean there are some things we simply do not recognise, or blank out, in everyday life. These specifically alter from person to person, however there will be things that happen in your life that you simply never know are there. Uranus helps us sense and acknowledge these things; the other points of view, the illogical and irrational elements to our reasoning; the detrimental habits we have, which stop us from achieving what we want to achieve.

Take a moment to look at how society has changed in the last two-hundred years, the industrial revolution and technological advancements, social attitudes and the information age. When you understand how much a piece of technology changes society or how something as simple as a TV show or film can radically alter our cultural 'schema', you will see the perspective of the Uranus Essence in action.

A fascinating dynamic to observe is when the Essences of Uranus and Saturn come together. Whenever you witness people with traditional or old-world morality speaking against modern ways, or when people, en masse, pull away from a once powerful organisation, this is Saturn (the traditional or once-accepted view) interacting with Uranus (the progressive approach). The two create divergence, as opposed to integration. This is an important partnership to bear in mind when a client needs to move on from some old way of doing things, but resists the new way as completely alien.

Saturn/Uranus together widen the incongruity, enabling you to repattern the old, whilst expanding the new.

NEPTUNE

Idealistic and compassionate, the Neptune perspective is one that inspires us to stand up for the rights or needs of others; be they human, environmental, animal, or circumstantial, etc. Whenever a person is compelled to express themselves for some greater cause, or feels compassionate towards something more than themselves, it is the viewpoint of Neptune at work.

This can lead to actions and opinions that are disconnected from the whole, however, for example; when people use bombs to fight for political or religious causes; when activists use arguments that are out of touch with the nature of things; when individuals sacrifice themselves for something that is not expansive or progressive in nature.

The illusion of good and evil, right and wrong, are a part of Neptune that are essential for many, yet define circumstances, attitudes and situations that can be limiting on higher levels. All things are definitions, some of which we place emotional value on. If the emotional values are compromised we tend to see this as bad or wrong in some way. Conversely, the bolstering of our emotional attachments feels good, or correct. Universally though, these are illusionary, transitory, and deeply personal (even when common in society) definitions of something far greater in power and omnipresence.

Nevertheless, we can work with Neptune to create illusion in times of need. For instance, when treating a person who sees nothing but pain and suffering, we can create hope or instil a belief of happiness. If the person then goes on to think this belief or feel that hope for long enough, it will become a reality for them (they replace one illusion for another that is more expansive). The essence is also excellent for people who takes things too literally, or are unable to understand the concept of a metaphor. Neptune enables illusion to play a part in the areas of life that are not as definitive or 'as they seem' to others.

PLUTO

The perspective of Pluto is intense and shocking to the way of all things; it is transformation and complete renewal. The Pluto Essence is power and self-mastery; it creates anew from what is obsolete, but in such a way as to be unrecognisable from what was. As such, Pluto is excellent when a person needs complete change; the initiation of total transformation. Remember that Pluto always works wonders and it does so in mysterious, unpredictable ways.

Pluto Essence can shift the viewpoint of those who are used to power and getting their way, to a place of greater balance; the domineering parent of an adult will begin to see the relationship more as equals; the aggressive manager becomes more receptive to suggestions from staff; an overbearing partner will learn to share in responsibility and decisions.

The essence will also help those without power to attain it for themselves, by cementing it into their perspective. This will never become all-encompassing power, but the power of equality. For Pluto is not of dominance, nor is it the essence of tyranny; it is the potent force that comes when two, equally powerful forces work with each other to create something between them. Pluto is synthesis and cooperation, even if the path is turbulent at times.

Wonderful when used for personal goals or business, the creation of a group, company, or project, Pluto is unconventional and slightly surreal in its approach. Perhaps the reason we never perceive the way it works is, because if we did, it would be too unbelievable to be possible in our reasoning.

Pluto brings truth to the surface, uncovers mysteries and offers clarity to where there was once enigma, though the essence itself is always intangible and mysterious in action. This is reflected in the psychological, cerebral layers of action that Pluto tends to focus on. Analytical, and at times, hyperconscious, this essence has a profound effect on the subconscious mind and levels of consciousness that need to be reached for through practice and deep, personal insight.

GAIA, THE MOON AND THEA

In Celtic Reiki there are three aspects that affect us more than most others, these are: Grandmother Sun, the Moon and Father Earth. The Sun (Sol) offers us life, she is like a mother to the Earth and all who are part of the Earth. The Earth is not only our home and the reason core of our physical existence, it is who we are on a physical level. The Moon has an immense influence upon us, from the balance of water to gravitational dynamics and many other unseen forces that constantly affect us.

We shall explore the nature of Sol in the next section and, in many ways, the essences of Earth are detailed throughout this encyclopaedia and have great relevance in every essence that is perceived through the human senses. To dismiss the Earth in a planetary perspective would be to leave out an important part of the whole, so in Celtic Reiki we use a trinity as our foundation...

Gaia, the Earth Mother and life-force of the Earth. The Moon; sister of the Earth. And Thea; the ancient brother that impacted the Earth, billions of years ago to create what we now know as the Earth and the Moon. It is common practice to separate the Moon and Earth as physical entities, however the union of the two as life-forces, combined with the force that created them offers us connection and reminds us that nothing exists in isolation—it is definition that forms an illusion of diversity and separation.

The trinity essence of Gaia, The Moon and Thea is life born through calamity, fire and destruction. For in the creation of the Moon and the Earth, both Thea and the old Earth came to the end of their existence and were reborn with the potential to create life. From two tiny planets, came something rare and precious: a planet that was exactly the size needed to retain a life-giving atmosphere and a satellite that regulates many of the essential forces on planet. This happened at exactly the right distance from the Sun at exactly the right time for the collision to be an act of creation, rather than destruction.

When we shift to the perspective of this essence, we are reminded that we were born in the dynamic of perfection—where everything is exactly how it needs to be for us to be here. At every step of the process the one thing happened for life to be viable. And not only life, but intelligent life that can connect to a vast consciousness that is higher than itself. This begs the question, did life just happen or did that consciousness create the environment for life to happen?

In Gaia we see consciousness; the Earth as an Eagle and as a tree and as a human. The Gaia aspect of this perspective is our Earth-self that perceives life as the Earth, yet separated by the illusion of being an eagle, tree, human, and so on. Gaia is the force that connects our physicality and Earth layers of consciousness. She is the benevolent and all-wise mother that gives physicality and takes it away. Yet, she always ensures that in pain there is some greater reward, some form of rebirth, just as she experienced from the death of her old selves.

The Moon aspect is mysterious and half-seen—we know the effects of the moon, but do not see what causes those effects. We know the moon is always there, but she is not always visible. The Moon is of the Earth and of Thea, just as we all are, yet she represents something beyond ourselves, something more. She is illusive and faraway, yet she is still part of us. Like a drumbeat that resonates in us all, reminding us that who we are is not only what we see and touch—some parts of who we are, exist beyond our perception and if we perceive with our inner-knowing, we will see the effects of these parts of us in the effects they have upon us and our world.

Thea is of rebirth; an ancient part of us that most people are unaware of, forgotten because the label that is used to define it is not the label of perceived importance. Thea is just as much a part of us as we are a part of Thea, yet our simple acceptance of the modern-day Earth means that most people never actually know who they are and how they came to be here. Thea reminds us that labels change, the solid world shifts in a slow, finite way, but the underlying core of who we are still beats within us.

THE
STARGATE
ESSENCES

STARGATE

The Stargate Essence creates a link between the Standing Stones and the Celestial Realm and is based upon the concept of standing stones being a gateway to other worlds, dimensions or layers of consciousness.

Originally based on the Stonehenge Essence, Stargate now incorporates Lay Lines and stone circles from all over the world. Its purpose is to provide what some may call an 'Astral Travel' experience that facilitates communication with other levels of consciousness (non-human intelligence). In other words, the Stargate helps us connect to and exchange knowledge with higher beings.

The Stargate is combined with a second essence; usually that of a constellation, star or planet which is known to have conscious intelligence associated with it. A selection of these is included in this section, although there are many thousands of other essences that could be Calibrated to as part of your Celtic Reiki Mastery adventure.

Activated as with any other essence, Stargate then creates a layer in which the secondary essence can be 'wrapped'. When used without a 'destination', the Stargate perspective is deeply healing and vibratory in nature—particularly suited to the creation of 'portals' and stone circles of your own—the Stargate is excellent when dealing with 'environmental modification' and the changing of physical anchors. This means that you can use Stargate by itself (or with any Celtic Reiki Essence), to treat your home, office, or any physical environment.

It was the Stargate Essence that eventually led to many of the Viridian Method philosophies, which focus on treating vast layers of physical and non-physical reality. In Celtic Reiki, however, the focus is much simpler in nature and consists of the two essences in tandem with each other (Stargate and destination essence).

SOL

When used as a destination for the Stargate Essence, Sol (Earth's own Sun) connects us to a vast and powerful consciousness. In many ways, the very attempt to define what this consciousness is, limits it greatly. Whether the consciousness belongs to other beings, some higher intelligence or the Sun herself is moot, because if you attempt to establish what or with whom you are communicating, you diminish its capacity and potential.

Whenever you or your client is in need of guidance or you want to add an element of profound sentience to your treatments, align with the Stargate perspective, followed immediately by Sol.

CERES

The Ceres Essence is very different in feel and perception to Sol, yet is strangely familiar. This essence tends to be experienced as 'individual consciousnesses' rather than the undefinable qualities obtained through Sol. In other words, there is distinct personality with Ceres. This personality is often described by Celtic Reiki Masters as a 'council' or 'official group' of beings that deliberate on challenges and offer their guidance. This wisdom seems displaced in time, as if beyond time, which denotes intelligence that is non-physical in nature.

TITAN

Titan is very different in feel and feedback from the previous destinations, for it hints at a civilisation, rather like that of humankind, but one that is to come, instead of one that exists in parallel to us. Indeed, cosmologists believe that when the sun expands to a specific level, the geology and chemistry of Titan could support intelligent life. Could this be the source of Titan's many voices? Whatever the source, the essence of Titan is cultural and social in perspective, giving the sensation of a vast and complex structure.

ORION

This constellation, destination essence is both powerful and wise. Symbolic of both the Roman legend of Orion and the Egyptian God Osiris, there are elements of these two cultures in the perspective of Orion who is fatherly in nature. The vulnerability of both the hunter Orion and the betrayed Osiris can be felt in the benevolent nature of this consciousness, which begs the question; does the essence come with cultural preconceptions of the constellation, or was the intelligence associated with Orion to influence the foundations of both these legends?

OPHIUCHUS

The perspective of Ophiuchus is also ancient and individual, as with that of Orion; one has a tangible sense of an individual, sentient consciousness with this destination essence. Ophiuchus is focused on success, achievement and the ability to excel in every moment of life. There is a deeply physical quality to this view that hints this perspective has been tried and trusted in the physical world, perhaps many millennia before we came to be here, perhaps at some point in the future, or even in this moment, right now.

PLEIADES

The Pleiades Essence has a certain level of motherliness, which could also be interpreted as an elder sister or aunt. The qualities of the Pleiadean perspective are focused on communication and alternative ideals. The entities that we connect to through the Stargate destination of Pleiades invite us to transcend ourselves, rather like a trusted relative teaches us to be more than we were in the past. Here, though, we are asked to go beyond an Earthly perspective of what we believe the world (Universe) to be and step into an unimaginable new way of sensing our lives and experiences.

Alpha Centauri & Proxima Centauri

This Essence is the perspective of three different stars: Alpha Centauri A, B, and Proxima Centauri. This trinity presents us with a viewpoint that some may call 'technological', though if you open up to the intelligences of this destination, you will see the wisdom is actually more balanced than is initially apparent. For this is not technology as we understand it, but the technology of spirit and thought; practical ways of developing frameworks and strategies to benefit our own lives and those of the people we meet along the way.

Barnard's Star

Our closest neighbour, the essence of Barnard's Star is so tangible, it is almost part of us and yet, it is very distant. It could be said that the beings connected to this destination are not of any reality that we can reach, or that they are so different from us, as to make little sense. Yet, our proximity in physical perspective has thrown us together in some way. An interesting, if slightly perplexing essence, which some resonate with more than others!

Sirius

The very first destination essence, Sirius is our connection to a group of entities that inspired much of the evolution of Celtic Reiki and subsequent therapies. The 'Lemurian' could be viewed as non-physical reflections of the solid world, wise and ancient beings that were once a part of the solid Universe, but became disillusioned with the world and its physical nature. In transcending their physical selves, they became beings of the light and left a trail of breadcrumbs for us to follow.

The Lemurian way is the most associated with EnergyLore of all perspectives and as such is often assigned to those who are not really in-touch with the 'real world'. Conversely, there is a reality in the 'seeded' information of the Lemurians that rings truer than most of our social and cultural ways of understanding the world.

The idea of 'seeded information' could be viewed as 'messages' woven into the fabric of the Universe at specific layers of intelligence and consciousness. When we expand to these layers, we can access this wisdom from our own perspective and make it our own. This not only provides us with greater wisdom, but also offers us a 'map' that we can use to Calibrate to the next layer of information.

This does seem to suggest the Lemurian knowledge is ancient (from the past), and whilst any physical remnants would be historical in nature, the wisdom is timeless and energetic, meaning it can be translated into relevant knowledge in any age or period of existence.

POLARIS

The directional opposite of Sirius, the Polaris destination connects us to a more 'Atlantean' perspective, akin to the shaping and geometric philosophies of the Volcanic South. Here, the way of perceiving information is more tangible, physical and connected to a modern, scientifically-orientated world. The Polaris Essence gives us a perspective that is parallel to that of Sirius, except the way we interpret it is more 'acceptable' or 'digestible' for people.

This could also be viewed as a difference in interpretation; Sirius is more inclined towards the right-hand brain and Polaris leans to the left. This makes Polaris focused and logical, direct and forceful. The Polaris perspective is individual and the definitions that create it are more rigid than the Lemurian way. This results in a propensity towards dogma and 'my way is the right way', rather than the perspective-driven view of Sirius. This can be very contractive and it can give us strength of conviction when we need to argue our case.

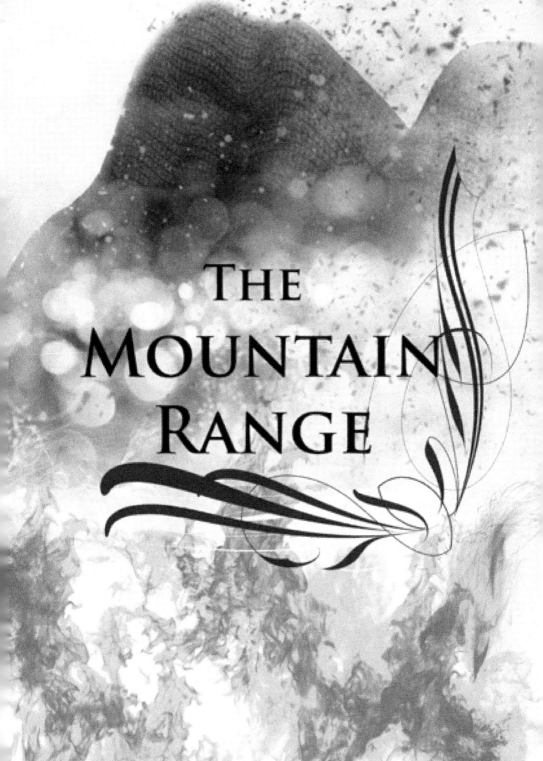

THE MOUNTAIN RANGE

THE
NORTHERN
PEAKS

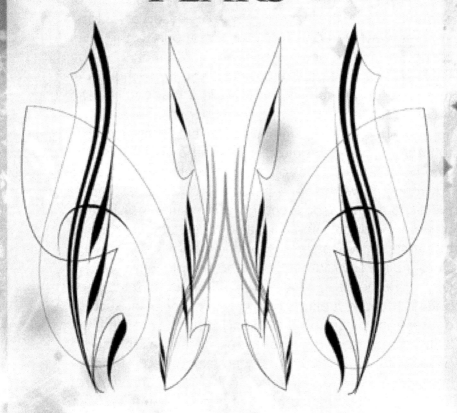

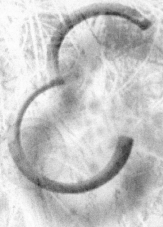

Schumann

The essence of Schumann is used to initiate the start of a treatment or harvesting. It activates the ever-shifting perspective of the Schumann Resonance, which is in continual flux. So, when employed in the harvesting of essences, Schumann basically filters out the 'background noise' of contrasting perspectives or attitudes. All the Earth's living creatures are very sensitive to the Schumann Resonance and react to its capricious nature, hence changing their own perspective in line with it.

Many humans have become disconnected from the Earth's natural resonance, however, and cannot understand why they have become dis-eased or feel lost in some way. By adjusting your vibrations to the level of the Schumann, you are basically reconnecting to the Earth. This is a valuable activity at any time, though in the harvesting ritual, you are ensuring that you gain an accurate sense of the viewpoint of the potential essence.

Therefore Schumann is a perspective to shift to when clarity is required. For example, the essence can be used outside of a treatment, or harvesting environment, whenever a person is 'out of phase' from the Schumann Resonance and this results in a feeling of unease, depression, anger and so on. Shifting to this essence will have a soothing effect on you, your surrounding environment, and the people in it.

Remember that the Schumann Resonance does not cause feelings of contraction or pain, such as depression, or anger. It is being out of sync with the Schumann that causes these feelings and aligning into phase with it will dampen any adverse effects. Modern humans, as a species, tend to be quite unaware of the natural rhythm; so do not tend to shift without encouragement. This usually comes via dis-ease, trauma, or with a nudge from helpful Celtic Reiki Masters!

PLANT HARVEST

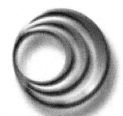

Used for the connection to and the harvesting of any perspective that is plant-based in physicality. The Plant Harvest viewpoint creates a 'focus' that is particular close to that of plants. This nurtures an understanding of plants and the experiencing of a closer connection to the way they perceive the world. As a very different perspective from our human outlook, we often need to strip away years of programming and sensory data to get close to the nature of plants; this essence was specifically designed for that purpose.

When you come to harvest a plant essence, the first thing you should bear in mind, is to inform the plant, tree, etc. what you intend to do, re-assure the plant that you will not harm it and ask for their permission. These seemingly trivial steps are in fact the most important activity in the whole procedure of harvesting plant vibrations.

Treat all plant-life with exactly the same respect as you would another person. Trees and shrubs have been treated with little, or no respect since the disappearance of the Celtic peoples and after centuries of being regarded as 'things', many are deeply mistrusting and suspicious of humankind.

It is so important to realise the intricate balance that exists between plant and animal species. In a physical sense we feel superior, as we can move and talk and create things, although on many levels, trees and plants are just as conscious as we are. Certainly the older trees are more knowledgeable about life, too!

The creation of a new essence involves no giving or taking other than time—just as a conversation does not involve us taking from another or them from us. However, the asking of permission could be seen as asking a person if it is convenient to talk. By treating each plant as an equal, rather than something to possess (or assume is there just to pander to our needs), we develop a global relationship with our plant cousins. We can learn from them, as they learn from us and we share our views, rather than entering into what could be called a domineering relationship.

Each time we connect with a plant, our perspective is in some way altered, and that alteration can be sensed by every plant we encounter subsequently. If you assume that you can harvest without taking time to respect the plant's time, it may affect future harvesting, as the plants you encounter may become unreceptive in reaction to 'another human' who disrespects them. However, by ensuring that you communicate your intent and ask permission, the plant will gladly share their insights with you and you will have made a friend for life!

This ethic is one that is at the spiritual heart of Celtic Reiki, for our way is about loving all things and being in complete harmony with the world around us. So when you propose to harvest the perspective of a tree, even though you are not physically taking from the tree, you should ask its permission first.

Once you have ascertained the receptiveness of the plant in question, centre yourself and shift to the Schumann Resonance, followed by the Plant Harvesting Essence. The method that is often best suited to plants is one of very intense focus, as this converges right in the heart of the plant's viewpoint. As you do this, you may feel a pressure or synaesthetic sensations (such as heat, cold, etc.) emanating through you.

As you continue, any synaesthesia is likely to get stronger and begin to centre on your hands, feet, abdomen or in your mind's eye. You can help the progression of the harvest by being open to it – and if necessary allowing yourself to move. (Some people report a pulling back, or spiralling motion, others may find their hands being pushed further apart, or a turning of their head. Always stay grounded if this happens to avoid falling over!)

This is the point where you define the essence, by specifying a name, symbol or another form of trigger. These are the parameters you will use later in treatment situations. If you are using a notebook, write down these details as soon as you have completed the harvest.

You should be aware when the harvest process has been completed the sensations will shift, either through a feeling of restlessness, a 'letting go', or just some sense that it has been done. At this point, thank the plant and wish it well. You may like to take some additional action as a token of gratitude to the tree. This could be bringing some natural fertiliser with you, a treatment or even a donation to an environmental charity.

Remember to make notes, including the time, date, plant type and any intuitive information, or synaesthesia effects you had during the harvest.

ANIMAL HARVEST

The Animal Harvest Essences directs our attention to the holistic perspective of any animal (including the human species!) and enable us to create essences of an individual or species. The focus of the resulting essence tends to be physically- or cerebrally-oriented, inasmuch as it is the viewpoint of the creature's physiology and psychology, as opposed to our own ideas or traditions of the animal. So, let us say you wanted to harvest an essence that represented the druidic nature of the stag. Here you would be advised to conduct a Concept Harvest, rather than an Animal Harvest, as you can instil a sense of the druidic tradition into the process. An Animal Harvest would most likely result in very different views and results.

As with plants, you should always maintain a respect for the animal you wish to work with, by explaining what you are doing and ask permission. Do bear in mind that animals react differently to plants and, whilst animals do tend to be more aware than humans, their sensitivity to Celtic Reiki is not as refined as that of plant species. So be prepared for the odd occasion when the animal will run off, or recoil when you start the harvest process.

The essences of Celtic Reiki cannot harm any living thing; conversely by using them, you may actually promote a healing environment for the subject, so harvesting is good for them. Without prior experience of Celtic Reiki, however, animals may just be uncertain of what is happening and prefer to retreat. You should be aware, when dealing with larger animals, or those with teeth and claws that they may want to get 'through you' in order to get away! You should always be prepared for unpredictability when working with animals and it is perfectly acceptable to wear protective clothing (or work at a distance) where necessary.

If you find certain animals just too daunting to approach, but still would like to create an essence, you can also use 'Concept Energy' to harvest a perceived or conceptualised perspective.

When harvesting the essence of animals, there will be many different experiences to deal with. So decide before you start whether you wish to harvest holistically or to focus on a certain aspect of the animal. A particularly useful perspective is unhealthy tissue, such as skin conditions, tumours, etc. as these can be used to help heal the issue on others.

MINERAL HARVEST

Minerals include such a vast range of subjects that each harvest situation you encounter will call for a different technique and it is often a case of taking each incidence as it is presented to you. Common mineral vibration collections you may wish to exercise are crystals, metal, rock, water, etc. To harvest the perspective of crystals, metals and loose rock simply hold the subject in your hand, then activate the Mineral Harvest Essence .

When you are harvesting crystal vibrations, remember that you are working with a living subject and therefore should explain your intent and ask permission. Crystals have a definite way of responding—if it does not hurt, or burn, you can proceed!

If you are harvesting from a huge amount of a mineral, for example a mountainside, beach, etc. just place your hands flat against the surface of the source. On the contrary, if you are dealing with a fragile, or minute mineral subject, such as a snowflake, or diamond fragment, simply place your hands over the source.

Water is of special consideration, for some particular types of water are seen to be healing (Chalice Well, Lourdes, etc.) and some can be detrimental to health (mineral, or radiation poisoning). Whenever you encounter a new source of water, you would be better to create a new essence rather than mixing or combining. Remember to ensure your own safety when dealing with water and other minerals that are detrimental to health. In this endeavour, always ascertain a correct identification of the mineral before handling.

ARTIFICIAL HARVEST

The main quality of this essence is a perspective of versatility, in conjunction with the ability to harvest many different sources. It is the best-suited perspective when creating essences for anything artificially made.

As with minerals, the possibilities of this category are so endless that individual situations should be tackled as they arise. You will harvest the energy of mobile phone in a very different way from a jumbo jet! For that reason, I shall leave the method up to you, suffice it to say that the Artificial Harvest Essence is extremely versatile and will help you to harvest almost anything!

Energy Harvest

This perspective will offer the best style of harvest for any form of energy from physical (heat, light, sound, etc.) to ethereal (spiritual energy, thoughts, etc.). Energy creates one of the most fascinating sources we, as therapists, can use. Homœopathic remedies of radioactive materials, sound and various coloured lights have shown us that there is a huge amount of scope here, especially when coming into contact with the modern dis-eases and trauma that we encounter as complementary therapists.

As energy can be intangible, the actual method of harvest is best decided upon in the moment or on an essence-by-essence basis. When writing your notes, remember to describe the details of the method of harvest and any extra information that is available about the energy itself. "Fire vibration collected from log and coal fuelled fire", "Light vibration from 60w tungsten bulb", and so on.

PLACE HARVEST

When harvesting places both in time and space, geographically, or by period, you can work with the Place Harvest Essence. This fascinating perspective can also be used creatively to shift towards viewpoints such as: areas of space (stars or planets) and places in time; so you can harvest the vibrations of historical events, such as the 'energy of a battlefield' to help those traumatised by war, etc.

The perspective of a place is a strange inclusion here, as energy exists beyond time or space and therefore, does not understand a 'place' as we do. However, places are definitions, like the physical labels we use for an amazing array of perspectives. Anybody who has experienced the healing peace of a church, or the invigoration of a cliff top, the atmosphere of a theatrical performance, or a concert, we tell you that places are not just physical locations.

It is usually a mixture of environment, people (or lack of) and other living things, motion etc. that synthesise to create the essence of a place. The Place Harvest Essence is similar to the previous harvest, though it has a greater focus on the surrounding physical area, rather than energy of pure definition.

When harvesting the essence of a place, you should try, wherever possible, to include in your notes information about the time and date, geographic location and you may find it helpful to make notes about the weather conditions, physical situation (people around, an so forth), and other physical factors that may have affected the harvest and resulting essence.

Microscopic Harvest

This essence is essential in the perception and harvesting in the perspective of both microscopic life and materials. It can be also be used when treating a person to scan for infection, or disease (cold virus, etc.). There are two types of microscopic perspective you may wish to harvest in essence form; those from microbes, such as bacteria, amoeba, parasites, etc. and that of the non-living; dust, and so forth.

It is important to consider whether you want to ask permission from the microbes you are working with. As these are some of the most important essences we can create, it is worth considering how you will personally work with the Microscopic Harvest Essence. One way to gain access to microbes without the need to consider 'permission' is to ascertain the availability of that microscopic agent as a homœopathic remedy (many subjects can be found this way, in all categories). This is a particularly useful method with illnesses such as HIV/AIDS, Herpes, and so on, as these are readily available from homœopathic pharmacies. Be aware, however, that the process of 'potentisation' would have been used to prepare these remedies.

FOR ADDITIONAL 'TRIGGERS', PLEASE SEE YOUR FURTHEST MOUNTAIN REALM, ONLINE.

THE
VOLCANIC
SOUTH

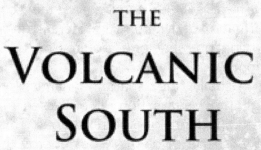

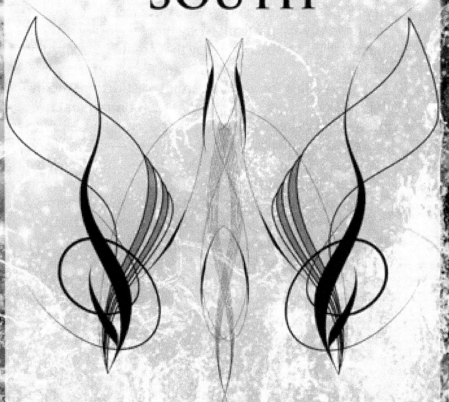

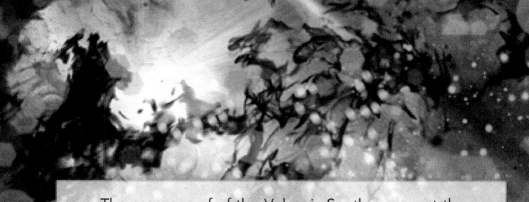

The essences of of the Volcanic South represent the creation of something solid and tangible, still in fluid form. These are the coming together, construction and formation of dynamics that increase in complexity, depending on what one requires for each, specific situation.

Usually, the 'shape' dynamics are formed through the visualisation of an essence projected and fashioned into geometric shapes. This does not create a 'shape of energy', but energy that creates results in a very particular way. For example, energy that acts like a cube or energy that creates a triangular outcome.

As this rather important distinction means that the energy is acting from a certain perspective, rather than having a physical shape, we can Calibrate to these perspectives of energy—the Shape Essences. Thus, Celtic Reiki Masters can choose whether they wish to shape essences through visualisation (The Three Mystics, mPowr) or simply trigger the essences included here. These contrasting approaches could be equated with the Lemurian and Atlantean perspectives of the Stargate Essences; with the Lemurian way being the use of perspective-based essences and the Atlantis method being one of mechanical steps to produce similar, yet distinct results.

The following descriptions have been kept to a minimum so that each Practitioner or Master can have their own experiences, based on their perspective of the essences, or the minute nuances of their shaping techniques.

THE LINK

The 'Link' is a basic shifting technique that creates a shared perspective, or link between you and your focus. You could look at this as being a simple connection between you; the connection consisting of whatever essence(s) you are working with at the time.

THE PULSE

The 'Pulse' expands upon the Link technique to generate a more elaborate connection that not only extends in every direction of perspective, but also produces greater force of influence.

THE SPIRAL

When we direct intent as a 'Spiral', it creates the effect of heightening the potency of the energy work. It is here that we begin to notice how visualisation does not create a shape in the physical environment, but instead, forms a perspective where energy results in the 'action' of the shape. For example, the Spiral is not a spiral in physical dimension, it is the perspective of a spiral.

THE ECHO

The 'Echo' is a little more complex, because as you Calibrate your perspective towards this essence, it Orientates back towards you. As this dual shifting of viewpoint takes place, there is an increase in the potency of the results obtained.

THE TRIANGLE

By working with this essence, we transition from one point to another, via the third point, therefore we create a style of energy that is best suited to problem-solving and resolving issues in a physical context. Energy shifts through both the 'focus' of the issue and 'resolution' of the issue, before returning to the original perspective as a solution.

THE CUBE

The Cube can be used in conjunction with essences to encapsulate and envelop, isolate or neutralise, and to assert/fix one's perspective. By working with the Cube Essence, you create definition that includes what exists within that definition and excludes everything else. Hence you wrap the focus of treatment or practice in the perspective of focused results in specific areas of awareness.

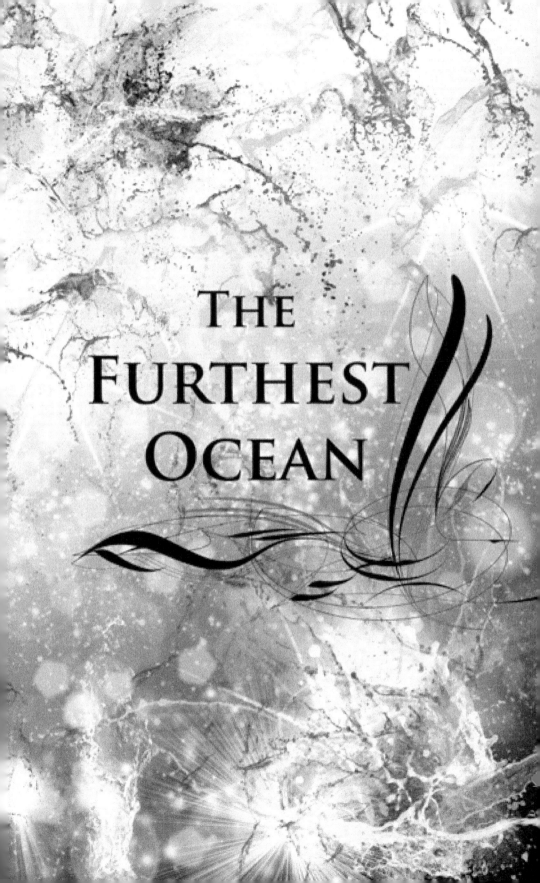

THE
FURTHEST
OCEAN

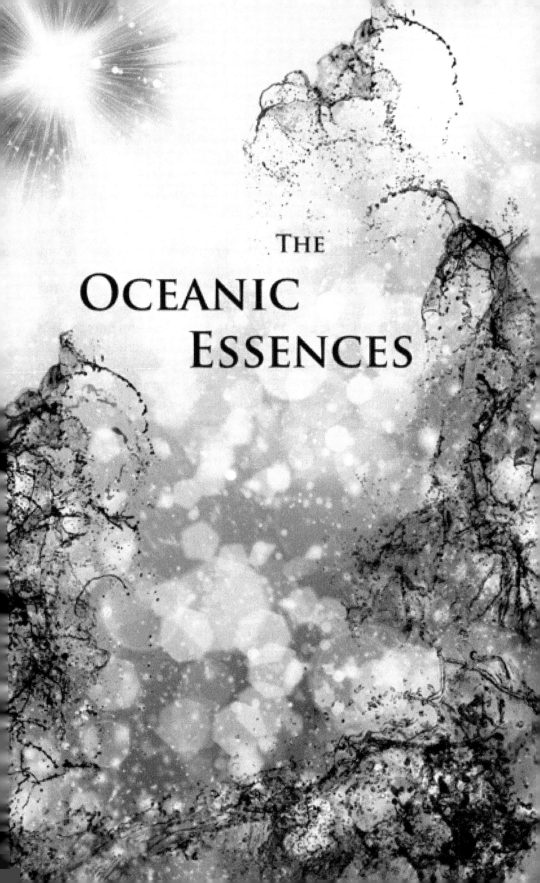

THE
OCEANIC
ESSENCES

THE ATLANTIC OCEAN

All the Oceanic Essences are associated with Mor and, to a certain extent, all share the same philosophies of deep truth and freedom from limitation and fear. Each Ocean of the world plays a slightly different part in the overall perspective of Mor, and this offers us the ability to alter and fine-tune our practices by adjusting to the different Oceanic Essences. As the Master Essence of the Furthest Ocean, Mor has an enigmatic quality that is somewhat more powerful that the Oceanic Essences, however these can make a valuable contribution to the treatments and practices that have specialist needs.

The Atlantic Ocean is a potent and forceful perspective that is expansive in dynamic. The Atlantic is increasing in size as each year the deep trenches at the bottom of the ocean push the Americas and Europe farther apart. As many of the Celtic lands border the Atlantic, this Essence has major influences on Celtic Reiki.

There is a powerful majesty and mystical fierceness to the perspective of the Atlantic; it is evolving, growing, and becoming more than it was. Therefore the essence has many characteristics of the one who strives to be and do more. There is ambition, hope, motivation and courage here, which can seem to be selfish and callous (particular if you stand in its path!). Nevertheless, this can be of immense value to the Practitioner or Master who feels that a dramatic or drastic shift is in the best interest of a client or student.

This essence is a wake-up-call to the major changes we face in our technological, modern lives. It represents, not only new or advanced knowledge, but also different approaches to coping with the learning of that knowledge. For example, the need to learn exponentially to cope with the amount of wisdom that the Information Age presents us with, rather than the old linear ways of learning. The truth of the Atlantic is a modern truth that requires a very unusual method of learning!

THE IRISH SEA

With such strong Celtic connections, the sea that lies between Ireland and Scotland/Wales, is perhaps the most closely associated perspective to the Mor Essence. May of the Celts would have looked upon this stretch of water, or fished from its depths. The Celtic Reiki Essence of the Irish Sea is a reminder of how the ocean adapts and changes whilst staying the same. The Irish Sea of modern times will look very much the same as it did two-thousand years ago, however the actual water that it is made of is very different now.

THE NORTH SEA

The North Sea touches the coasts of Ireland and Scotland, encompassing the Shetland and Orkney Islands and extending towards Norway. Whereas the Irish Sea is a reminder of transition and change, the North Sea is more mysterious and ancient; there is an element of permanence to this perspective.

Embracing both the Celtic and Nordic traditions, this essence has a tendency to feel quite solemn and isolating in nature. It could be described as an austere reverie or the foreboding before a ferocious storm! This heightens Mor's perspective of fear and the majesty of the sea's power.

THE ENGLISH CHANNEL

The busiest shipping channel in the world, the English Channel flows between England and Continental Europe. Here we begin to sense the influences from the Gallic Celts in a rich, 'warm' perspective that is both passionate and exuberant. As a region that never becomes very deep, this essence has a leaning towards the shallow qualities of Mor, such as the wisdom that exists near the surface and the common-wisdom of people. Hence we can reacquaint ourselves with the profound knowledge that we know, but tend to forget when held in the grip of emotion.

THE NORWEGIAN SEA

The Nordic Influences reach their greatest levels in this essence, which brings the Furthest Ocean and Standing Stones Realms together, giving a more fluid feel to those fixed perspectives. This viewpoint is aggressive in nature, creating powerful healing, a somewhat brutal wisdom, and the idea of honour through death. There is a blending of attitudes that combines the Warrior with the Adventurer, the Alchemist with the Wise One and brings them all together; therefore this essence is the best facet of Mor to work with when carrying out a practice across mystics.

THE MEDITERRANEAN SEA

This beautiful Mor Essence is unlike the other Celtic Oceanic Essences, for it is warm, nurturing, giving and inviting. This is not to say the other essences are cold and ungiving, it is just that the Mediterranean Sea Essence has these traits in abundance. The rich and vibrant perspective, makes colours brighter and light seem more refractive. It brings all the wild enthusiasm of the sea on a summer's day and pours them into any treatment or practice. This brightly-hued, ostentatious view of Mor is also the 'least-Celtic' of these initial Oceanic Essences, however there is a much closer link than those that follow...

THE ARCTIC SEA

The frozen seas of the Arctic represent the place where Mor becomes solid and fixed. Here the Master Element of the Elemental perspectives becomes most like Pridd and, whilst they are never exactly the same, here Mor shows many of the longer lasting qualities of the Earth. Therefore, at times when you wish to anchor a treatment using Mor, the Arctic Sea Essence provides a way of attaining all the qualities of Mor, but 'frozen' in physicality for as long as they are needed.

The Pacific Ocean

The Pacific perspective is vast and expansive, yet its dynamic is one of contraction. Now this is often seen as a 'negative' or unwanted result, however contraction is necessary for the solid world to exist. Without contraction, how would anything that exists at an expanded level ever make it into the physical world. The mechanism which allows higher wisdom, inspiration, spirituality, creativity, and advanced knowledge to exist in the physical world is contraction—these higher levels of experience contract into physicality. Have you ever wondered why we feel angry when dealing with behaviour that is childish or primitive? It is our invitation to contract to the level of people who are functioning on those layers of experience. When we do not contract, those people will often drift away or start to expand to our level, depending on the distance between us.

The Pacific Essence helps us to contract into denser layers of physicality, without the need for some emotional 'carriage' that feels horrible. By using the Pacific Essence, we close the gap between ourselves and those who function at a more physical level of perception. This enables us to communicate a higher wisdom, using a more traditional approach that is easier to understand.

This, in turn, enables others to expand to higher layers of spiritual awareness and wellbeing, without the rather messy 'game' of emotional ups and downs that we so often choose to partake in.

When perceiving from the Pacific Ocean perspective, remember that people will not suddenly start to think exactly as you do—they will continue to think as themselves, but simply from a higher layer of perception. This means that personal choice and preference are preserved and we get to revel in the wonder of individuality and uniqueness that makes us who we are. For more on the expansion and contraction of perspective, please see 'The Three Mystics of Celtic Reiki' (mPowr).

The Indian Ocean

The Indian Ocean brings diversity to the Mor Essence and provides us with a richness in the practice that would otherwise be missed. In Western culture, we often mix and match philosophies to suit our needs. Usui Reiki methods are often based on Indian Medicine, rather than Japanese traditions, Celtic traditions are often viewed with modern prejudices, and so on.

The Indian Ocean perspective creates continuity and congruity in this blending of cultures and beliefs. So, if you want to work with different philosophies as part of your Celtic Reiki Mastery, the Essence of Indian Ocean will offer you a means of integration and will also improve the results you achieve.

The Red Sea

The Red Sea perspective, like the Indian and Pacific Oceans, brings a blending of cultural influences and traditional methodologies together, to form a diverse and congruent therapy. With much of the Red Sea Area saturated in ancient ways and religions, the view of this essence enables us to produce a degree of flexibility in dogma and outmoded beliefs. This not only helps when working with those who are dogmatic or prescribe to beliefs that contract modern society, it also works wonders when we are trying to understand the root message of ancient words.

The Caribbean Sea

The Caribbean Sea perspective brings contrast to the Mor Essence when compared with the previous three essences, there is a similarity in their viewpoints. The Caribbean brings a modern feel to the Mor Essence, progressive and transformative, it gives us the ability to revitalise old ways and to totally redefine what was into what can be. Hence, the ancient is highlighted once more, but this time in a very modern perspective.

THE
COLOUR
ESSENCES

Red (Red Light, Including Pink and Infra)

When shifting to the perspective of Red, the Master or Practitioner can also specify different shades to alter slightly the focus of any practice. These shades are: Crimson, Scarlet, Vermillion, Maroon, and Pink. The effects of these essences will all tend to present the results detailed below, however, by specifying the difference in tone, effects will alter slightly honing your results.

Crimson often offers results of deeper resonance that are physical in nature, whereas Scarlet has a greater emphasis on sexuality, Vermillion on the intellectualisation of this perspective (more thought-based) and Maroon, creates a combination of Red and Blue perspectives. Pink is much softer and emotionally driven, giving the most contrast to all the tones in the Red viewpoint.

Red is traditionally associated with the physical world, solid and material layers of being, money and security. The psychology of Red presents a colour of passion, blood, anger and aggression that invigorates and arouses. Restaurants use Red as a very attractive colour that draws people in, but one that can only be tolerated for a short time, thus encouraging people to eat and leave quickly!

This is similar to the Red perspective in Celtic Reiki, as the essence tends to be one that is either combined to soften the effect or which is used briefly in treatment. Shifting to the Red viewpoint will bring attention to finances and the ability to support oneself and one's family. The essence tends not to be one of manifestation, but of focus. This means that the application of the Red Essence in treatment will highlight issues surrounding money, security, etc. so that other essences can be triggered to create greater results.

The Red perspective also increases our sense of passion and vitality; motivating and spurring us into action. The Red Essence increases our ability to act in the world, get tasks completed, results achieved, and lowering workload. Red is fantastic when a person feels lacking in enthusiasm for something they once felt passionate about, or helps support those who are dedicated to a cause.

ORANGE (ORANGE LIGHT)

The colour of the physical body and sexuality, Orange is traditionally employed to increase physical energy, sexual prowess, charisma, and sporting ability. The psychology of Orange as a colour is very similar to that of Red, though for many it is not as initially attractive, whilst a few are completely drawn to Orange in any shade.

The essence of Orange in Celtic Reiki has offered interesting feedback in the past, for in many incidences the essence follows the traditional perspective. Conversely, some feedback conveys a much more spiritual message in the Orange perspective, which is not surprising, as it is a sacred colour in several cultures.

The perspective of Orange can therefore be used to boost stamina and ability when conducting physical exercise, playing sports, etc. It also help maintain the willpower to complete physical challenges, like marathons, triathlons, etc. The Orange Essence is of paramount importance when helping others to foster a greater awareness of healthy eating and nutrition. Helping those who are on eating regimes, such as no sugar, low fat, no gluten, and so on.

The other facet of the Orange perspective tends to be much more spiritually-centred, although a body-focus is often commented on in feedback. Here the cycles of the body are viewed as part of a greater scheme; the holistic nature of the body, where our health reflects our spiritual level of attainment. The body becomes a physical manifestation of the mind and spirit, rather than the old notion of 'housing the soul'. Therefore, we see our bodies as extensions of source, instead of receptacles.

This integrated view of the physical flowing from the non-physical, is continued beyond the self and into the world; bringing the concept that we are all a part of a complex dance of source energy, sparks that momentarily offer glimpses into a magnificent solid world of matter and mechanics, where a single thought can create miracles.

Yellow (Yellow Light)

The Essence of Yellow is very similar to sunlight, yet without the cooler blues, violets and the more aggressive reds and oranges. It therefore provides the vibrancy and invigoration of the Sun without any of the other effects. Hence, the Yellow Essence is a wonderful perspective whenever we are working with darkness and stagnation; be it environmental, personal or social.

The places where people do not tend to go because they usually end up feeling drained or otherwise intimidated; people who are draining or upsetting to be around; group meetings or wider social dynamics that create contraction, rather than an expansive result; these are ideal candidates for Yellow, however be aware that if you encounter any of these, it might be self-treatment that you require, for this same perspective must exist at some level of your own being for you to perceive it externally.

Yellow is also an excellent essence for depression, offering revitalisation and a boost to a person's vibrancy. When a client has no sense of self or lacks confidence, when they put themselves down a lot or will not stand up for themselves, the Yellow perspective will heal their ego in a balanced and harmonious way, as well as motivating and invigorating.

GREEN (GREEN LIGHT)

The perspective of Green has long been associated with love, harmony and natural beauty, as well as being viewed as a very healing colour. In certain forms of Asian spiritually and homoeopathy the heart chakra is often viewed as being green in colour and thus, green is also said to be remarkably active in this area and connected physiological systems.

It is no surprise that feedback from the use of the Green Essence surrounds areas of treatment such as healing the inability to accept love, or feeling unworthy of love, overcoming guilt & resentment, mending of broken hearts and harmonising the mind and emotions. The perspective of Green shifts us to the level of a deeper emotional-cerebral relationship with nature. Green soothes the heart and lungs and is excellent for asthma or respiratory dis-ease, thymus nourishment and as an immune system booster.

One of the most enchanting elements of the Green perspective is that of the innate sense of peace and tranquility it offers. Psychological research has long presented the idea that the colour green calms the mind and emotions, encouraging our minds to conjure up memories of green pastures and sunlit woodland. These beautiful links are also seen in treatment and when used in spiritual practices. Masters, practitioners and their clients often report a tangible sense of being 'in nature' or 'outside', when they speak of interactions with the Green Essence.

The Green perspective, as with all the colour essences, can be blended with other colours to alter the results obtained in treatment or practice. For example, the combination of Green and Blue will create Turquoise, whilst Green and Red form the Brown Essence.

Blue (Blue Light)

Blue light was harvested from sunlight refracted through a prism, and has a deep, integral resonance with the throat, voice and creativity. Traditionally, blue is a colour associated with water, air, and travel, whilst also being revered in mineral form in the stones of Lapis, Aquamarine, and Sapphire.

The Blue Essence reflects much of the traditional philosophy inasmuch as it nurtures creativity and artistic expression, in conjunction with helping us to express what we need to express. Blue is wonderful at empowering us in the finding of our emotional and intellectual voice, paramount for people wanting to teach their spiritual truth to others.

This essence is cooling and soothing to the mind and emotional self. It alleviates a fear of flying and, with Aquamarine, relieves seasickness. Other physical aspects of this essence include healing dis-ease of the throat & thyroid gland, respiratory difficulties of the upper windpipe and can be useful when a system 'contracts'—Asthma, Raynaud's Syndrome, muscular spasm, etc. Blue stimulates spiritual creativity, connects thoughts and forms a bond between the 'conscious self' and the higher self.

INDIGO (INDIGO LIGHT)

The Indigo Essence has a rather profound effect on the Pineal and Pituitary glands, which shifts our perspective to a much higher range of perception. This viewpoint is somewhat intuitive, psychic, and possesses many skills associated with higher spirituality.

The important factor to remember here is not the symptoms or end results that manifest from the Indigo perspective; it is the act of shifting to a perception where activities are recognised that is important. In other words, a person may display greater psychic awareness in their words and actions after a treatment using Indigo, but it is how they can evolve themselves using this expanded perspective that is the real gift of this essence.

This perspective is one of deep insight and meditation, thus, will helping one to reach heightened levels of awareness. The benefits are not only spiritual, but mental as well, for the Indigo Essence accelerates learning and improves adaptive thinking ability. This translates not only to better problem-solving and higher levels of intelligence, but also immense creative ability, unconventional thinking and peripheral thought abilities.

Positioning oneself from the viewpoint of Indigo enables a person to reach the most expanded perception of self, before the definition transcends the self; in other words, when you see yourself through the eyes of Indigo, you are looking at the greatest level of expansion you can be, before becoming more than the self. Take one more step and you lose self-definition and understand the self to be more than a person and more than a person can comprehend.

VIOLET (VISIBLE & ULTRA)

As we shift beyond the Indigo perspective, to that of Violet the beliefs, ideals and ways of humankind lose cohesion and become nonsensical. Merely a series of physically-oriented definitions that are used to make the nebulous more tangible. We begin to realise that we are only what we think we are and that reality is what we believe it to be. Gradually we shift further and further into the Violet Essence and the illusion becomes clearer the closer we get to the Violet perspective.

Violet has similarities with the Cernunnos perspective, for whilst the Violet Essence is included as part of the Orientation programme (unlike Cernunnos), it takes time to learn and master the Violet Essence in a way that cannot be taught. When Calibrating to Violet, the Apprentice learns a foundation, which acts as a catalyst for change. It is this that will help the student to learn and eventually facilitate the changes necessary for a greater understanding of the Violet perspective. The paradox of the Violet Essence is that as it strips away the illusion and delusions of humankind, we can only sense what we have striped away within ourselves. In the most accurate, human perception of the Violet Essence, there is absolutely no connection with the self as a human being. We literally lose ourselves!

This means that for every human parameter we retain when shifting to the Violet perspective, we are one parameter away from actually knowing the truth of this essence. The actual use of this essence does not make one any less human; it simply propels our perspective to a place beyond human perception. This means that to get the benefit of Violet, we need to be more than human, by shedding our human limitations. This is one of the most challenging aspects of spiritual growth and also one of the most rewarding. When a person attains the perspective of Violet at any integral level of beyond-human recognition, they glimpse all things from all perspectives and experience a moment of utter understanding and total bliss. One joyous experience that will stay with them forever.

MAGENTA

Magenta, along with Cyan and Yellow is a secondary colour that still has great relevance for us, but is often forgotten. (Yellow is sometimes viewed as a primary colour, especially in pigment form.) As the perspective of intense creativity, the Magenta Essence connects us to a very primal source of creation, such as that of our ancestry and as a celebration of the Earth. Colours become more vibrant with a shifting towards the Magenta perspective, sounds more vibrant; even tastes and smells are richer in texture.

This intense connection to the Earth brings with it the overwhelming creative passion that is often sensed in artists and masters of a craft—from the great painters and poets, to actors and musicians. If ever you have witnessed a performer completely lost in the rapture of a song, or a writer in true flow, you will have glimpsed the power of the Magenta Essence: a power that can be recreated with a shift to the perspective of this essence.

CYAN

Cyan is an interesting colour, because we cannot actually see it! Whenever we look at the colour cyan in the physical world, the structure of our eyes creates a very slight variance in the precise tone and vibrancy of the colour. We can experience true cyan in synaesthetic response— some people 'see' cyan when listening to certain sounds, others when working in an altered state or with energy. This essence is based on this actual colour, based upon synaesthesia cyan, rather than 'physically reproduced and seen' cyan.

The Cyan Essences helps us to speak with a spiritual voice that inspires and changes lives. Like Magenta, it unleashes a profound creativity that can be transmitted through art or performance, however this perspective is spiritual (Universal or cosmic) in nature, as distinct from Earth-centred.

WHITE

These final two essences can be seen as polar opposites—complete absorption of light (Black) and complete reflection of light (White)—however there is also a contrasting approach, in which one is the absence of the other. White is the presence of light, however black is merely a lack of light (because the light is absorbed). In this instance, these essences are not opposites, but simply contrasting.

The perspective of white is reflective, stark and direct. It is the essence of purity, though this can denote being under the spotlight or unable to take action for fear of blemish. Under the gaze of the White Essence, nothing can hide—all is known—and anything that stands in the face of this essence casts a shadow. This can be pretty overwhelming, but does force one into resolution, albeit without pleasantry!

White is all-knowing and encompasses all things, yet it lacks definition and the experience of those things in isolation; therefore it must become something other than White to grasp what it is made of.

BLACK

The Black Essence is the unknown perspective, the one that needs to be brought to the surface, highlighted, and investigated to be known. Like White, it is all things, yet from this viewpoint these are all unknown and waiting to be discovered. The Black Essence is adventure, curiosity and the need to discover what is beyond our current knowing.

The Black Essence absorbs and repatterns, so is excellent at removing what is no longer needed or wanted. It soaks up the energy of habitual thoughts, contractive emotions, or limiting beliefs and rather than hiding them, the essence transforms them into something wonderful, simply waiting to be discovered.

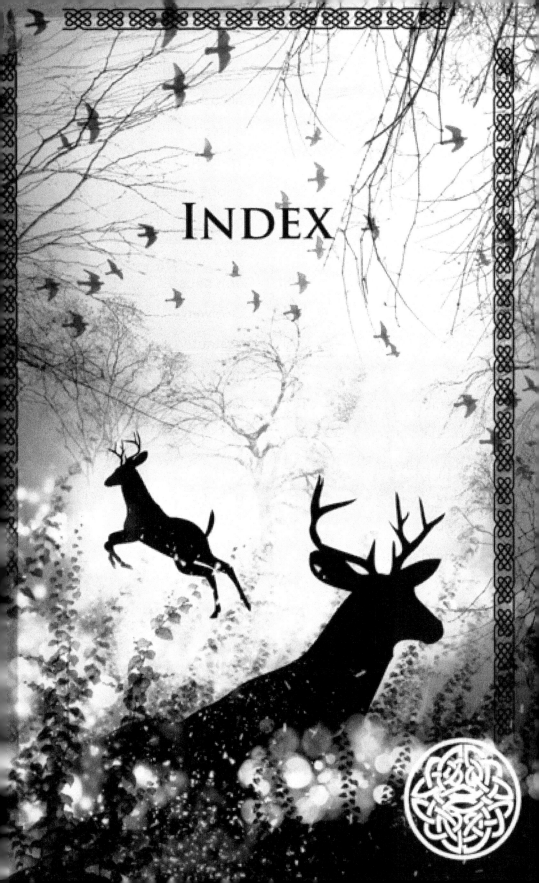

Index

Elm	107	Huathe	54
Emerald	175	Ifin	93
Energy Harvest	228	Indian Ocean	242
English Channel	239	Indigo	249
Eoh	156	Ing	162
Eolh	157	Ioho	31
Eucalyptus	117	Iolite	179
Fearn	41	Irish Sea	238
Fehu	161	Iron	177
Forseti	165	Isa	160
Foxglove	124	Jera	160
Freja	166	Jet	173
Frigg	168	Jupiter	205
Gaia	210	Kenaz	154
Garnet	180	Koad	144
Gemini	190	Labradorite	173
Ginger Root	128	Laburnum	125
Ginseng Root	128	Lagu	159
Gold	178	Lemurian Seed Crystal	184
Gort	76	Leo	192
Green	247	Libra	194
Gyfu	155	Lilac Tree	119
Haegl	157	Lime	114
Hemlock	124	Link	233
Hornbeam	115	Liquorice Root	129

Raido	154	Straif	83
Red	244	Sugar Maple	113
Red Sea	242	Sycamore	106
Rhiannon	133	Tan	142
Rhywtawel	100	Taranis	134
Rose Quartz	170	Taurus	189
Rosewood	121	Teak	121
Ruis	86	Thea	210
Sagittarius	196	Thurisaz	154
Saille	45	Tinne	61
Salt	181	Tir	158
Sapphire	174	Titan	215
Sarsaparilla Root	128	Tree of Heaven	118
Saturn	206	Triangle	234
Schumann	222	Turmeric Root	129
Scorpio	195	Uilleand	89
Sigel	157	Unhewn Dolmen Arch	146
Silvanus	137	Ur	24
Silver	178	Uranus	207
Sirius	217	Uruz	161
Skadi	167	Vanilla Orchid	127
Smoky Quartz	172	Venus	203
Sol	215	Violet	250
Spiral	233	Virgo	193
Stargate	214	Walnut	120

Other Celtic Reiki Books in the Home Experience:

This book is part of the Celtic Reiki Mastery Home Experience from mPowr—to enrol visit the Official Celtic Reiki Website at www.celtic-reiki.com.

The Adventurer's Guide
The Three Mystics
The Master's Companion
The Realm Master's Almanac
Realm Master: Secrets (The Sacred Wisdom of Celtic Reiki)

Discover the **Bedtime Stories of the Woodland**, now available from mPowr Publishing: the enchanting tales from the Celtic Reiki Mastery Home Experience within a single VAEO. Read the stories, hear the narration*, and interact with the characters*. Experience the wonder of the Realms anew…

* When used in conjunction with your smart phone or camera-enabled tablet device.

Audio Programmes from the Author:

Synaesthesia Symphony IV: The Chorus of Creativity
Synaesthesia Symphony V: The Harmonies of Health
The PsyQ Orientation

For further information about Celtic Reiki and The Celtic Reiki Mastery Home Experience please visit:

www.celtic-reiki.com
www.mpowrpublishing.com

Lightning Source UK Ltd.
Milton Keynes UK
UKOW06f1417121117
312604UK00004B/81/P